Researching Dysl
Multilingual Settings

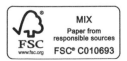

MIX
Paper from
responsible sources
FSC® C010693
www.fsc.org

COMMUNICATION DISORDERS ACROSS LANGUAGES

Series Editors: Dr Nicole Müller and Dr Martin Ball, *University of Louisiana at Lafayette, USA*

While the majority of work in communication disorders has focused on English, there has been a growing trend in recent years for the publication of information on languages other than English. However, much of this is scattered through a large number of journals in the field of speech pathology/communication disorders, and therefore, not always readily available to the practitioner, researcher and student. It is the aim of this series to bring together into book form surveys of existing studies on specific languages, together with new materials for the language(s) in question. We also have launched a series of companion volumes dedicated to issues related to the cross-linguistic study of communication disorders. The series does not include English (as so much work is readily available), but covers a wide number of other languages (usually separately, though sometimes two or more similar languages may be grouped together where warranted by the amount of published work currently available). We have been able to publish volumes on Finnish, Spanish, Chinese and Turkish, and books on multilingual aspects of stuttering, aphasia, and speech disorders, with several others in preparation.

Full details of all the books in this series and of all our other publications can be found on http://www.multilingual-matters.com, or by writing to Multilingual Matters, St Nicholas House, 31–34 High Street, Bristol BS1 2AW, UK.

Researching Dyslexia in Multilingual Settings

Diverse Perspectives

Edited by
Deirdre Martin

MULTILINGUAL MATTERS
Bristol • Buffalo • Toronto

To Leo and Olivia with love

Library of Congress Cataloging in Publication Data
Researching Dyslexia in Multilingual Settings: Diverse Perspectives/Edited by Deirdre Martin.
Communication Disorders Across Languages: 10
Includes bibliographical references and index.
1. Dyslexia. 2. Second language acquisition–Research. 3. Language and languages–Study and teaching. I. Martin, Deirdre (Deirdre M.), editor of compilation.
RC394.W6R47 2013
616.85'53–dc23 2013023034

British Library Cataloguing in Publication Data
A catalogue entry for this book is available from the British Library.

ISBN-13: 978-1-78309-065-5 (hbk)
ISBN-13: 978-1-78309-064-8 (pbk)

Multilingual Matters
UK: St Nicholas House, 31-34 High Street, Bristol BS1 2AW, UK.
USA: UTP, 2250 Military Road, Tonawanda, NY 14150, USA.
Canada: UTP, 5201 Dufferin Street, North York, Ontario M3H 5T8, Canada.

The policy of Multilingual Matters/Channel View Publications is to use papers that are natural, renewable and recyclable products, made from wood grown in sustainable forests. In the manufacturing process of our books, and to further support our policy, preference is given to printers that have FSC and PEFC Chain of Custody certification. The FSC and/or PEFC logos will appear on those books where full certification has been granted to the printer concerned.

Typeset by R. J. Footring Ltd, Derby
Printed and bound in Great Britain by the Lavenham Press Ltd

Contents

Figures and Tables

Figures

Tables

Contributors

Jean Conteh is Senior Lecturer in the School of Education at the University of Leeds, UK. She worked as a primary teacher and teacher educator in multilingual contexts in different countries for many years and, since 1987, has worked as a teacher educator in West Yorkshire, UK. She completed her PhD in 2001, investigating the factors which contributed to the success of pupils from minority ethnic backgrounds in multilingual primary schools. Since then, she has published many books, chapters and articles about multilingualism, education and social justice, and she continues working with primary teachers and students. Address: School of Education, University of Leeds, Leeds LS2 9JT, UK, email: J.Conteh@leeds.ac.uk.

Gad Elbeheri is Associate Dean of Foundation and Academic Support at the Australian College of Kuwait. He is an expert providing consultancy to the Center for Child Evaluation and Teaching (a leading non-profit centre in Kuwait which combines research and practice on specific learning disabilities across the Arab world). He is also the United Nations Development Programme's Technical Director of its the Early Learning Challenges and Disability Project. An applied linguist who obtained his PhD from the University of Durham, UK, he has a keen interest in cross-linguistic studies of dyslexia and other specific learning difficulties and their manifestations in Arabic. Address: Associate Dean for Foundations and Academic Support, Australian College of Kuwait, PO Box 169, Qortuba, Kuwait, email: g.elbeheri@ack.edu.kw.

John Everatt is Professor of Education at the University of Canterbury, New Zealand. He received his PhD from the University of Nottingham and has lectured on education and psychology programmes at universities in the UK (Wales and Surrey) as well as in New Zealand. His research focuses on literacy acquisition and developmental learning difficulties, particularly dyslexia. Current work focuses on relationships between literacy and language, for example how variations between scripts might influence literacy learning across different language contexts, including those involving multilingual learners. Address: College of Education, University of Canterbury, Private Bag 4800, Christchurch 8140, New Zealand, email: john.everatt@canterbury.ac.nz.

I-Fan Su is an experimental psychologist who studies cognitive processes involved in communication at the Division of Speech and Hearing Sciences at the University of Hong Kong. Her particular interests lie in visual word recognition, impaired language processing in Chinese (developmental and acquired dyslexia and hyperlexia) and applying electrophysiological (EEG/ERP), behavioural and cross-linguistic methods to the investigation of cognitive processes. She is a member of the Laboratory of Communication Science at the University of Hong Kong. Address: Laboratory for Communication Science, Faculty of Education, Meng Wah Building 8F, University of Hong Kong, Hong Kong, email: ifansu@hku.hk.

Carol Goldfus is Senior Lecturer at Levinsky College of Education, Tel Aviv, Israel, and head of the Adam Research Centre for Language Abilities and Multilingualism. She received her doctorate from the University of Birmingham, UK, and a postdoctoral fellowship from the Multidisciplinary Brain Research Center at Bar Ilan University, Israel. Her research focuses on the reading comprehension of underachieving pupils with language-related disabilities who are unable to succeed in academic settings. She specialises in literacy acquisition and metacognition with adolescents with difficulties. In teacher education, she is developing the field of educational neuroscience. She is a member of the executive committee of the International Academy for Research in Learning Disabilities (IARLD). Address: 28 Shear Yashuv Street, Jerusalem, Israel 97280, email: goldfus@netvision.net.il.

Bobbie Kabuto is Assistant Professor of Literacy Education at Queens College, City University of New York, USA, where she teaches courses in the areas of early language and literacy, bilingualism and biliteracy, and language and literacy in the elementary years. Her research interests include reading and writing in multiple languages, early bi/literacy, socially constructed identities, and language ideologies. She currently works with families of struggling beginning readers and writers. Her research examines the ways in which schooling discourses frame socially constructed identities and how and why families support or challenge these identities in the home. Address: Elementary and Early Childhood Department, Queens College, 65-30 Kissena Blvd, Flushing, NY 11367, USA, email: bobbie.kabuto@qc.cuny.edu.

Judit Kormos is Reader in Second Language Acquisition at Lancaster University, UK. She is the coauthor (with Anne Margaret Smith) of the book *Teaching Languages to Students with Specific Learning Differences* (Multilingual Matters, 2012) and a coinvestigator in the project Dyslexia for Teachers of English as a Foreign Language, sponsored by the European Commission. Her research interests include the psycholinguistics of second language acquisition and second language speech production. Address: Department of Linguistics and English Language, Lancaster University, Lancaster LA1 4YL, UK, email: j.kormos@lancaster.ac.uk.

Deirdre Martin is Senior Lecturer in the School of Education, University of Birmingham, UK. She has been involved in researching and teaching multilingualism and language disabilities throughout her academic career. Her particular interest is in multilingual language disabilities, and literacy practices and skills in multilingual contexts where there are low literacy skills and dyslexia. She has developed masters and doctoral teaching programmes in this field. Research methodologies and methods of creating knowledge are a fundamental aspect of her research interest. She has been involved in national and international research studies in multilingualism and language disability. Address: School of Education, University of Birmingham, Edgbaston, Birmingham B15 2TT, UK, email: d.m.martin@bham.ac.uk.

Gavin Reid is an independent educational psychologist based in Vancouver, Canada. He is a registered psychologist in the UK and in British Columbia, Canada. He was Senior Lecturer at Moray House School of Education, University of Edinburgh, from 1991 to 2007 and Visiting Professor at University of British Columbia. He wrote and developed the first masters course in dyslexia in the UK in 1993. He is a director of the Red Rose School in Lancashire, UK, and has made over 650 conference and seminar presentations in 68 countries. He has 28 books in print in teacher education, dyslexia, literacy, learning styles, motivation and classroom management. Email: gavinreid66@gmail.com.

Maria Rontou has been a teacher of English as a foreign language (EFL) at Greek state primary and secondary schools for seven years and worked in English schools for one year. She holds a BA in English Language and Philology from the University of Athens, an MA in English Language Studies and Methods from the University of Warwick, UK, and an EdD in Language Studies from the University of Birmingham, UK. Her academic interests include teaching EFL to students with dyslexia, inter-collegial collaboration, computer-assisted language learning and English language teaching (ELT) methodology. She has published articles on inter-collegial collaboration, differentiation for students with dyslexia and teaching EFL. Address: 2

Xenofontos St., Loutraki 20300, Greece, email: mariarontou720@hotmail.com.

Richard L. Sparks received his EdD from the University of Cincinnati, Ohio, USA. He is currently Professor at the College of Mt St Joseph in Cincinnati, where he teaches courses in reading, learning disabilities, assessment and research. His research interests are foreign (second) language learning, reading disabilities and hyperlexia. He has published numerous papers in both native language and foreign (second) language journals. He also has a private practice in which he conducts psycho-educational evaluations and consults with professional organisations. Address: College of Mt St Joseph, 5701 Delhi Road, Cincinnati, Ohio 45233, USA, email: richard_sparks@mail.msj.edu.

Carol To is an Assistant Professor in the Division of Speech and Hearing Sciences at the University of Hong Kong and a speech and language pathologist. Her research focuses on the assessment of and intervention in speech and language disorders in children, including speech sound disorders, autism spectrum disorders and developmental language disorders. Address: Laboratory for Communication Science, Faculty of Education, University of Hong Kong, Hong Kong, email: tokitsum@hku.hk.

Anastasia Ulicheva is a psycholinguist who studies cognitive aspects of normal and impaired language processing (aphasia, dyslexia). Specifically, she is interested in mechanisms that underpin skilled reading in Russian as well as the acquisition of literacy in typically and atypically developing Russian children. She uses behavioural, eye-tracking and cross-linguistic experimental methods to investigate the cognitive processes involved in language processing in healthy and clinical populations. She is currently pursuing a PhD at the Division of Speech and Hearing Sciences and is a member of the Laboratory for Communication Science at the University of Hong Kong. Address: Laboratory for Communication Science, Faculty of Education, Meng Wah Building 8F, University of Hong Kong, Hong Kong, email: ulicheva@hku.hk.

Brendan Stuart Weekes is an experimental psychologist who studies cognitive processes in communication. He investigates memory mechanisms in normal and impaired language processing (aphasia). He uses cognitive models of language processing to guide this work on reading, writing and speech production, and an experimental approach to study cognitive processes, including behavioural, brain imaging and cross-linguistic methods. He is also a clinical psychologist working with adults and children with communication disorders caused by dementia, dyslexia and poor reading comprehension in Indo-European and Sino-Tibetan languages. He is Professor and Director of the Laboratory for Communication Science at the University of Hong Kong and Convenor of Communication Disorders. Address: Laboratory for Communication Science, Faculty of Education, Meng Wah Building 8F, University of Hong Kong, Hong Kong, email: weekes@hku.hk.

Acknowledgements

My appreciation, thanks and gratitude to the following people:

For the invitation to contribute to their series with this edited volume and for their generosity and encouragement in all manner of ways – Nicole Müller and Martin Ball.

For creative scholarship in researching literacy, literacies and dyslexia in multilingual settings and their generosity in contributing to this volume – Jean Conteh, Gad Elbeheri, John Everatt, Carol Goldfus, I-Fan Su, Bobbie Kabuto, Judit Kormos, Gavin Reid, Maria Rontou, Richard Sparks, Carol To, Anastasia Ulicheva, Brendan Weekes.

For enthusiasm and indexing – Helen Bilton.

For encouragement and support and their incredible work in multilingualism – my colleagues in Mosaic, Centre for Research in Multilingualism, University of Birmingham, Marilyn Martin-Jones, Angela Creese, Adrian Blackledge and Maggie Kubanyiova.

For the terrific editorial and production process – Anna Roderick, Sarah Williams and Ralph Footring and the entire team at Multilingual Matters.

For creating Multilingual Matters publications and establishing multilingualism as a field of publication – the late Mike Grover, and Marjukka Grover and Tommi Grover.

Introduction

Deirdre Martin

Introduction

When planning this volume, I considered whether the notion 'dyslexia in multilingual settings' formed a field of study. I mean by a 'field of study' a body of knowledge that is constituted by sets of nested and symbiotic relationships across concepts, theories and analytical frameworks. The relationship between higher-order conceptualisations of knowledge and the practices of enquiry that create the knowledge constitutes the 'DNA' of the discipline. My question is: what do the various disciplines involved in studying dyslexia share with regard to conceptualisations of dyslexia phenomena? Do they share analytical frameworks for the interpretation of data, and if so how? Strong contenders as field-of-study candidates would be the disciplines of educational linguistics, cognitive and neurological psychology, as well as sociolinguistics and anthropology. Yet they each have distinct, and arguably incommensurable, ways of generating and interpreting evidence. Positivist approaches engage technical skills in their methods of data collection and analysis, while ethnographers have practices of enquiry that are interpretative and dialogic in nature.

Analyses of the nature of literacy studies through a model of overlapping disciplines (e.g. Rassool, 2002) often omit references to literacy difficulties/dyslexia and multilingualism. The few existing studies of dyslexia in multilingual contexts illustrate a 'bounded' approach to this area, where discipline structures and analytical frameworks make it difficult for theoreticians to engage with each other (for discussion see Martin, 2009). This chapter discusses an agenda for further research with a view to moving towards more inclusive interdisciplinary study. Bearing in mind that there is an epistemological purpose to educational research, namely to contribute to our knowledge of teaching and learning in practice (Hymes, 1981/1968, in Van der Aa & Blommaert, 2011: 5), the chapters in this volume reflect contributors' awareness of practice-oriented application of research to pedagogy and assessment in dyslexia studies in multilingual settings.

This volume has three aims. The first is to present, through specially commissioned chapters, current approaches to researching dyslexia and literacy in multilingual settings across disciplines and methodologies (these approaches are geographically and historically situated in the political 'west'). A second aim, addressed in this introductory chapter, is to draw on concepts and analytical frameworks of a more critical nature that suggest other interpretations of existing research discourses about dyslexia in multilingual settings. Critical analyses reinterpret pre-theorised notions of diversity as 'a multiplicity of factors' to reveal stark prejudicial social practices in contexts of dyslexia in multilingual settings. A third aim is to signpost directions for future research, towards a critical reconsideration of current understandings of dyslexia in multilingual settings, with a view to foregrounding the potential for interdisciplinarity.

The final section of this chapter sets out the organisation of the volume and the content of the chapters. The first three sections discuss key areas in the studies in this volume: literacy and literacies, dyslexia, and multilingualism.

Literacy and Literacies

Street (1984) redefined the field of study of 'literacy' by identifying two distinct conceptualisations: *literacy* and *literacies*.

Literacy is a theorised concept for a set of skills around print: orthographies and logographies in reading, writing and spelling and other scripts. These skills are conceptualised as cognitive, and, once learnt, are understood to be 'autonomous' of context (i.e. can be applied across contexts). This understanding of literacy skills continues to dominate most educational contexts in curriculum learning, assessment and intervention. Theories about literacy skills address development, pedagogies, motivation and cognitive processing, among others including dyslexia. The analytical frameworks that inform empirical studies of literacy and dyslexia tend to be normative and comparative (for respective examples of such framework, see Chapters 1 and 2 of the present volume). These frameworks are further discussed in the next section.

Literacies, by contrast, are conceptualised as social practices around print and texts which are embedded in social contexts, such as writing minutes of a meeting, texting or using libraries. Street further theorised the notion of literacies in two analytic frames: literacy practices and literacy events, where literacy events are instantiations of socially and culturally situated literacy practices (Street, 1984). In other words, literacy events are 'those occasions in which the talk revolves around a piece of writing' (Heath, 1983: 392). Literacy practices are social practices related to or with texts (e.g. purchasing online, using religious texts, tweeting) and literacy events are specific occasions on which people interact around print or screen (e.g. reading a story, discussing an individual education plan, hymn singing). New Literacy Studies (New London Group, 1996) have taken the concept of language and literacies further, to include modalities beyond talking and print (Kress & van Leeuwen, 2001). Multimodality is based on the assumption that meaning is made through the many means – modes – that a culture has shaped for that purpose (Kress et al., 2005: 21). Multimodal literacies include photos, signage, wall displays, a piece of writing, a drawing and children's early markings with pencils and crayons.

In her ethnographic work with multilingual children in homes and schools in London (UK), Kenner (2000) studies children's 'literacy worlds' at home and in their local community. Taking a sociolinguistic and interpretative approach, she presents literacy learning in school through an engagement of parents, children and teachers working together to build on the understandings gained from home. Multimodal resources such as computers, drawings and writing afford both literacy learning in English (the language of school literacy skills) and multilingual literacy learning through international networking resources. In her study Kenner showed how multilingual literacy learning is embedded in, and grows through the use of, social resources (see Chapters 7 and 8).

Ethnographic studies of learning literacy, skills and practices in contexts of learning needs and difficulties are comparatively rare (e.g. Flewitt et al., 2009; Kliewer, 1998; Lacey et al., 2007; Trueba, 1988). It is even more difficult to find published studies that conceptualise research into multilingual literacy learning in contexts of dyslexia through this lens. A powerful and unique study by Rodriguez (2005) looked at language and literacy practices of Dominican children with special needs in New York City. She examined the multilingual lived experiences of children's and their families' practices across home and school, illustrating and analysing the experiences of disjuncture between home and school language and literacy practices, not least the experiences of literacy practices in special educational provision. The absence in the present volume of a commissioned chapter based on the ethnographic study of dyslexia in a multilingual context reflects the paucity of research available in this area (and the need for more).

Dyslexia

Dyslexia is widely understood as a noticeable difficulty with literacy skills, particularly reading. These difficulties can occur in adulthood following brain damage (see Chapter 5). Most research, though, is conducted in educational contexts and, reflecting this, the majority of chapters in this volume are concerned with dyslexia in children. Developmental dyslexia refers to children's difficulties learning literacy skills despite unexceptional development in other regards and with typical educational experiences. Dyslexia in children is usually constructed with normative and comparative measures of literacy skills learning, which in turn reflects discourses of educational research, as well as education policies and practices (see Chapters 1–4 and 6). In educational research and practice, the performance boundaries of developmental dyslexia are difficult to distinguish from 'common or garden varieties' of reading and writing difficulties (Savage, 2004; Stanovich, 1994). There may also be difficulties with forms of notation other than orthography, for example numeracy. Social and emotional well-being may be impaired by the experience of difficulties in literacy learning (see Chapter 2). However, fuzzy boundaries are reflected in alternative terminology for the needs expressed by those with such learning difficulties. Take, for example, specific learning difficulties (SpLD) and, in many parts of the world, learning disabilities (LD). Whatever term is used, literacy skills difficulties are usually discursively constructed as difficulty rather than need, with respect to the interference in school learning.

Understandings of a biological basis for dyslexia

There is general agreement that we do not have a genetic predisposition for written language (orthography, logography), although we do seem to have one for spoken language. Rather, written language is culturally shaped, with biological and cognitive bases (Frith, 1997). However, research studies do suggest that problems in learning literacy skills may have hereditary features. In the absence of genetic predisposition, what may be inherited are particular biological, neurological and cognitive capacities that are insufficiently recruited or recruited in such ways as to give rise to literacy difficulties. Discourses in the dyslexia literature construct these recruitment problems as 'deficits', while alternative discourses construct them as 'partial recruitment' of biological, neurological and other resources (Savage, 2004). However, the bottom line is that, over decades, the substantial biological/ neurological literature – for example, localisation studies in the temporal lobe and areas of the brain cortex, speed of response to visual/written and auditory/spoken language – has remained inconclusive about the *causal* roots of developmental dyslexia (Savage, 2004). As with spoken language, we draw on (sufficiently or otherwise) biological, neurological and cognitive capacities to learn to communicate through scripting and other modalities.

Historically, medical research constructed developmental dyslexia as brain-based. Although neurological studies continue, this discourse is less influential, as cognitive psychological approaches to studying information processing are now preferred for this language-related disability. However, the situation is different for acquired dyslexia. The importance of localisation studies is more obvious when dyslexia results from specific brain damage. This research approach was associated with studies locating centres of brain activity, for example Wernicke's and Broca's areas with speech. With computational advances, neurological investigations use neuro-imaging to scan and record neurological activity during literacy skills activities, to produce more sophisticated mapping of networks of neural activity. More recent still, computational modelling is used to test scientific models or hypothesises against empirical research and clinical literature. These methods are used particularly if it is difficult to test the science in reality. This method is used to predict how the brain manages multilingual visual orthographic or logographic scripts across languages (see Chapter 5): are there routes and pathways for each language?

The dominant discourses in researching developmental dyslexia and acquired dyslexia are still 'within the head' discourses, that is, cognitive psychology, psycholinguistic and neurological discourses (see Chapters 1–5). While dyslexia is widely constructed as an individual's difficulty, there are historical, social and cultural issues that need further consideration in understanding dyslexia.

Mass education and literacy for all

Dyslexia was identified in the late 19th century in England, at a time when literacy skills became more accessible to the wider populace both through schooling and socially, with the increase in books and libraries. More recently, the requirement of 'education for all' encourages measures of population literacy levels to be included in national statistics, particularly in developing countries, as an indicator of universal education. The quality of high-stakes testing has been critiqued. So what had been skills for a small, elite, educated class worldwide became available to all through mass education. In the UK and most countries, the learning of literacy skills happens in contexts of schooling, and so difficulties in learning literacy skills, including dyslexia, become a construct of schooling; education practices therefore need to be considered along with individual difference and disability.

Now, in the early 21st century, we are positioned at an equally momentous and propitious time to look at social engagement with new digital literacies and changing literacy practices (Barton & Lee, 2013). Moreover, new multilingualisms in literacies are being forged through new ways of blending language resources in print and on screen. With some exceptions (e.g. Smythe, 2010), few new literacy practices are incorporated into official schooling pedagogies for literacy skills, other than highly directive, computerised, monolingual writing and spelling programmes. Here is an opportunity for innovative interdisciplinary studies on, for example, the performance of dyslexia in digital literacies among multilingual urban youth and in the inclusion or exclusion of writers with dyslexia. In the same vein, interdisciplinary opportunities are afforded for dyslexia that results from brain damage.

The pedagogic making of ability and dyslexia

One line of critical argument advances the notion of 'ability' as a construct of schooling: 'The concept of differential "ability" is very much a product of the establishment of mass schooling' (Kress *et al.*, 2005). Kress and colleagues, in a study of three urban secondary schools in England (2001–03), identified the main features of schooling that contribute to forming this construct: these included a prescribed national curriculum, frequent testing, and pedagogy that matched teacher expectations of pupils' ability. The level of control exercised through curriculum pathways and forms of assessment creates a homogeneous profile of educational response across diverse learners. A corollary of 'authorised knowledge' about literacy skills in a national curriculum, with a national literacy programme, taught through prescribed pedagogy from the early years of schooling, is the increased likelihood of failure among multilingual students learning the language of schooling, and among students who learn literacy skills differently. There are also increased pedagogic challenges for their teachers. But so long as learners who appear to have dyslexia are provided with appropriate educational support, such as specialist intervention programmes (e.g. Hatcher *et al.*, 2006; Torgesen, 2005, 2009; and Goldfus in Chapter 3 of this volume), they can acquire literacy skills to the point where they can achieve at school.

Monolingual performance and monoliteracy have become privileged in most education systems. Moreover, literacy skills in the language of school are privileged over literacy skills in home or community languages (see Chapters 7 and 8). Where multilingualism and multilingual literacies are ignored and monolingual literacy skills are seen as having greater value, literacy difficulties and dyslexia become a priority for assessment and intervention as special educational needs.

Low language skills and print difficulties

Of serious import here is that, in multilingual settings, dyslexia may go unidentified, under the shadow of developing the language of schooling, for example English as an Additional Language (EAL), or learning the curriculum for foreign languages. That is, low language proficiency is used to explain difficulties with print. Additional language learning is often confused with learning difficulties for several reasons: limited language support, low valuing of languages other than the dominant school language, limited assessment protocols in the non-dominant languages, and use of the dominant language in testing protocols with linguistic and cultural biases against the students (Artiles *et al.*, 2011; Cline & Shamsi, 2000).

Claims of 'unfairness' in identification processes (e.g. Peer & Reid, 2000) have received responses from two quarters: technical/cognitive and critical ideological. Professional bodies, such as the British Psychological Society (1999), and researchers in the cognitive psychological and psycholinguistic traditions, have engaged with assessment protocols that aim to be more 'culture fair' and to have fewer linguistic biases, as well as with assessments in minority languages (e.g. Martin *et al.*, 1997) (see Chapters 1, 2 and 4). This approach continues to construct educational difficulties largely through a 'medical model' where the problem is located in an individual with deficits, who requires 'fixing' through intervention (see Chapter 4).

The other avenue of response takes a critical sociological approach to interpret the multiple interlinked social, linguistic and discursive processes that generate inequality. It is mentioned here though there is little research as yet following this approach and applying it specifically to dyslexia in multilingual settings. There is, however, some research that focuses on inequality created by the discourses that circulate in settings of linguistic diversity (Artiles *et al.*, 2011).

Disproportionality

Disproportionate representation of school students across social categories of ethnicity, language and ability in special education is evidenced in local and national statistics (e.g. Artiles *et al.*, 2011, in the USA; Lindsay *et al.*, 2006, in the UK). Studies in the USA and the UK show that disproportionality is an important site of study that reveals either too many or too few students identified with special educational needs.

In the UK, the statistical analysis[1] has revealed that students from particular multilingual communities are *under-represented* in the category of 'dyslexia/SpLD' (Lindsay *et al.*, 2006). Pupils of south Asian origin who have a heritage in the Indian subcontinent and pupils of Chinese origin are *less likely* than white British pupils to be identified as having specific learning difficulties, or moderate learning difficulties, or autistic spectrum. Lindsay *et al.* (2006: 4) report that:

> The literature suggests that this could be because of difficulties in disentangling learning difficulties from issues associated with English as an Additional Language (EAL) and therefore work is needed to assess whether these children's needs are being met appropriately or whether their EAL status is leading to an under-estimation of the nature and severity of cognition and learning needs.

A partially similar profile is reported in the US literature (Artiles *et al.*, 2011). In the USA, as in the UK, multilingual learners with language-related needs/difficulties are likely to be under-reported. By contrast with the UK, in the USA multilingual minority students are, though, over-represented in special education, with alleged cognitive learning difficulties. The quote above from a UK report offers an explanatory comment from a technical perspective that obfuscates the main issue.

There are also more subtle indications of discriminatory practices. EAL learners in secondary school have been placed in literacy support classes designated for learners with special educational needs. The rationale is 'educational rationing' due to lack of resources (Gillborn & Youdell, 2000).

Together, these studies are strong evidence in support of the view that special education placement is less about learners' biologically based needs and more about the cultural practices of education professionals.

Intersectionality

In both the UK and the USA, monolingual and monocultural education policies generate a discriminatory profile of disability for specific groups of students. Critical analysis holds that monocultural and monolingual conceptualisations of social relationships and formations in society across ethnicity, class and gender give rise to prejudice and oppression. Crucially, it is the interrelatedness – intersectionality – of social categories of identity that gives rise to discriminatory behaviour. Lindsay *et al.*'s report reveals that monolingual and monocultural education policies generate greater social and educational inequality. However, some of the text fails to state this clearly. Analysts in the USA recognise that the monolingual and monocultural orientation of educational policy towards English is a means of replicating inequality in education. They advocate that it be recognised as such and challenged (Artiles *et al.*, 2011). Critical research could examine the discursive construction of the social categories of ethnicity, class and gender, and the ways in which these are linked with measures of language and literacy skills, specifying how they give rise to practices of inequality by education policy makers and policy implementers (see Chapter 6).

Multilingualism

Three different ways of conceptualising multilingualism and literacy/ literacies shape discussion in this volume: language and literacies as bounded entities, as unbounded fluid and variable practices, or 'translanguaging', and as a continuum.

Language and literacies as bounded

Structural and bounded understandings of languages underpin mono-lingual education policies, and inhibit interactional flow across languages, and the development of multilingual identity and self (see Chapters 7 and 8). For example, English (including English as an additional language) is the prescribed language of pedagogy in the UK and elsewhere, and in many other countries English as a foreign language (EFL) is the language of instruction from primary school onwards. In these contexts, engaging multilingual talk and literacy skills in pedagogies in mainstream classrooms can be problematic on several levels. When educators do not share students' languages it is likely that some multilingual students will be perceived as having learning needs and difficulties even when this is not the case.

Language as unbounded: Translanguaging

A critical alternative analysis to boundedness in multilingual research is unboundedness. Fragmentation of language as a structural notion in talk and informal writing (e.g. texting, digital literacies) is taking place among speakers who share language codes (Duchêne & Heller, 2012). Translanguaging (Garcia, 2009) is a term that describes the multiple discursive practices in which multilingual speakers engage to make sense of their multilingual worlds. Speakers develop 'flexible multilingualism' (Blackledge & Creese, 2009) and 'pick and mix among the languages they know at various levels' (Li Wei, 2010). While including code-switching practices, translanguaging is more extensive, in that it covers other multilingual practices, such as literacies and literacy skills. Garcia (2009) posits that multilingual speakers tend to blend the language resources within their shared repertoires in rapid, informal conversational styles.

Translanguaging in pedagogy has been studied in learning spaces other than formal schooling. For example, in community language schools in the UK, multilingual teachers and students draw inclusively on their linguistic resources, spoken and written, in curriculum teaching and learning (Creese & Blackledge, 2010). In segregated classes for learners who are deaf or hearing impaired in Sweden, teachers and students translanguage across spoken and signed languages, as well as written, visual and media modalities in the course of a lesson (Bagga-Gupta, 2012). Multilingual spaces are interactionally created (Li Wei, 2010) and translanguaging disrupts artificial allocation of language medium to spaces in the curriculum.

Bilingual language and literacies as a continuum of resources

In a critical anthropological paradigm, Hornberger and Skilton-Sylvester analyse bilingual language and literacies as a continuum organised by attributed power and privileging practices (Hornberger, 1989; Hornberger & Skilton-Sylvester, 2000: 96). For these researchers, literacy is an axis for distribution of power (Hornberger & Skilton-Sylvester, 2000). Their framework shows how learners are either constrained or enabled in their biliterate development. The more their learning contexts allow them to draw on all points of the continua, the greater are the chances for their full biliterate development. This model offers several levels of analysis for biliteracy development, across aspects of context, media and content, and within each aspect there is a continuum mediated by power and privilege. A further axis of power concerns privileging 'readers' over 'non-readers', which, in this model, refers to those who are excluded from access to literacies due to gender, ethnicity or poverty. However, although not necessarily intended by Hornberger and Skilton-Sylvester, it could also refer to those readers marginalised as having dyslexia-type difficulties and language learning disabilities (Martin, 2009: 107).

Diverse Perspectives on Researching Dyslexia in Multilingual Settings

A number of challenges face researchers involved in contemporary studies of dyslexia in multilingual settings. First, there is the challenge of generating knowledge in genuinely interdisciplinary ways. Second, there is the challenge of engaging in multilingual research practice, for example in research teams with team members of different cultural backgrounds, and speaking different languages. In such research teams there are likely to be power asymmetries which need to be acknowledged in democratic and reflexive ways (Martin et al., 1998). Third, there is the challenge of working ethically and maintaining critical awareness of social inequalities between groups speaking different languages. Researchers need to consider their stance (Cameron et al., 1992): are they doing research on, for, or with speakers of minority languages?

The following discussion offers a critical lens on the diverse research perspectives in the chapters in the volume. Where possible, it points to the potential for interdisciplinary approaches to researching particular aspects of dyslexia – both developmental and acquired – in multilingual settings.

Assessment

Normative and comparative practices involving testing are prevalent in researching dyslexia in aspects of literacy skills. Some testing procedures have transferred to educational practice and become assessment tools for children's performance for educational placement. Students with literacy difficulties/dyslexia at school are likely to be referred for diagnostic assessment with a battery of tests. Standardised assessments developed in research often have assumptions and protocols that 'presume that examiners are neutral conduits of prespecified items to which examinees respond with correct or incorrect answers reflecting individual level of ability' (Maynard & Marlaire, 1999: 171). A strand of research by Maynard and Marlaire (1999: 171) 'examines an interactional substrate in the testing sequence between examiner–examinee'. These researchers argue that the interactional substrate reveals scaffolding-type performances which clinicians depend on to obtain access to measurable, quantifiable abilities. That is, the 'mistakes' in the testing procedure by both clinician and child, which may not stem from inabilities or incompetencies, indicate interactional competencies. The authors conclude that 'bad testing' (that is, transgressions of the protocol) can be informed by good reasons to reveal children's interactional abilities. This approach to noticing the interactional substrate would inform pedagogy with children and adolescents with language-related disabilities, including dyslexia, in assessment regimes. It also informs dynamic assessment.

Dynamic assessment (DA) is suggested (see Chapter 1) as an alternative to testing regimes for phonological awareness. DA can, through its teaching/learning method, identify difficulties in learning aspects of language. At the same time, the method identifies language learning potential by appraising learners' responsiveness to specifically modified language interactions (e.g. for EAL and multilingual language disabilities see Hasson *et al.*, 2013; Peña & Gillam, 2000). A DA approach to phonological awareness and literacy skills with multilingual children who have dyslexia would afford more insight for subsequent pedagogy intervention.

Tomasello's (2003: 28) work on language development as a process of enculturation proposes two important characteristics of language learning through social meaning making: *intent to communicate* and *pattern finding*. That is, language development is motivated by intentions for social meaning making through a search for patterns in language making. The development of literacy practices and skills is probably motivated in similar ways. Yet there is an imbalance in researching both avenues in contexts of dyslexia. As with language difficulties, cognitive psychology and psycholinguistic research for the last 30 years have focused particularly on pattern finding as a central feature of learning reading, writing and spelling in English and other languages. Studies investigate abilities of learners to find patterns in tasks of phonological awareness and phoneme–grapheme correspondence. While this method seems diagnostically effective in differentiating students with literacy skills difficulties and dyslexia, the absence of meaningful communication needs further consideration. Pattern finding on its own holds little meaning for participants, particularly those with difficulties finding the patterns. Further, the method has been adopted across languages and orthographies without due consideration for the cultural perspective. Taking up a suggestion made by Everatt and colleagues in Chapter 1, a novel application of Tomasello's ideas would lead to research on learning literacy skills for understanding and meaning making through DA. This approach would offer new knowledge in an under-researched aspect of dyslexia in monolingual and multilingual text settings.

Interdisciplinary approaches are suggested in neurological research too. Recent studies of remembering in contexts of old age from a sociocultural perspective (Middleton & Brown, 2005) indicate both the necessity of, and the productivity that would follow from, interdisciplinary research on learning in contexts of neurological ill health and decline. There are few studies using this method with multilinguals or speakers of languages other than English. One suggestion for an innovative, interdisciplinary approach to acquired dyslexia could consider generating new knowledge that involves neuro-imaging people with brain damage or neurological ill health as they engage in multimodal practices, for example talking about old, personal photographs, in monolingual and multilingual contexts.

Timely and Future-oriented Research

We are on a faultline of new literacy practices. Already we are being thrown into a new world in which the arenas for literacy are no longer institutional in nature, that is, at school or at work. Digital devices have carried literacy practices onto the streets and around the globe in the hands of multilingual readers and writers. Literacy practices are becoming far more demotic and anarchic, and at the same time more meaningful to practitioners. New ways of researching are necessary for those of us who are concerned with investigating dyslexia in the new types of literacy events and practices that are cropping up in our contemporary multilingual, multicultural, multimediated global society. This way of researching must be malleable and light on its feet; it must be critical of previously prescriptive and prejudiced discourses that applied to a more monolingual, monocultural and monocommunicative world.

Researchers must ask: how do we research literacy skills difficulties and dyslexia in the context of these changing literacy practices and within the new communicative order? What will interdisciplinary dyslexia research, theory and practice look like in the multilingual settings of this new world? How can dyslexia research be responsive and relevant in this world? Critical interdisciplinary perspectives on researching dyslexia practices in multilingual settings are needed and researchers need to engage with this new world or risk being left behind.

The Chapters

The specially commissioned chapters gathered here showcase specialist knowledge and research approaches within the fields of multilingual literacy/literacies and dyslexia. They reflect distinctiveness of knowledge within and across disciplinary identities. Four main approaches to researching bi/multilingual literacies and dyslexia are presented: sociolinguistic, cognitive, neurolinguistic and pedagogic. Multilingualism is researched in contexts where English is a prescribed school and curriculum language, contexts where community languages are taught in school, contexts when foreign languages are included in the curriculum and, finally, contexts where a child's multilingual development in the family home language and school language is the main concern.

The first four chapters present studies of cognitive approaches to dyslexia in multilingual settings. The first two chapters present a cognitive methodology for the assessment of dyslexia in English, Arabic and foreign language curriculum contexts. The third chapter is concerned with a cognitive approach to a pedagogic intervention programme in English as a foreign language (EFL) for adolescents aged 16–18, in secondary school settings. The fourth chapter offers a critique of cognitive approaches to researching dyslexia in contexts of EFL.

The last four chapters introduce alternative methodologies. Chapter 5 presents a computational modelling methodology to investigate two hypotheses about multilingual reading in adult dyslexia. The sixth chapter is an organisational ethnography concerning the management of dyslexia needs in schools. Chapters 7 and 8 do not focus on dyslexia at all. Rather, they present Street's (1984) conceptualisation of literacies and literacy practices in research practice, taking different ethnographic approaches to multilingual literacy practices in classroom and home settings, from a sociolinguistic perspective.

In Chapter 1, John Everatt, Gavin Reid and Gad Elbeheri explore the literature around the problematic of assessment aimed at identifying dyslexia in bilingual learners. They comment on the under-representation of bilingual learners with dyslexia and provide an analysis of the inadequacy of cross-linguistic assessment procedures. They show a concern for cultural fairness with regard to assessment materials in the language of schooling, often English. The writers take a comprehensive view of the cognitive bases of literacy skills and cognitive-related difficulties in dyslexia.

In Chapter 2, Richard Sparks reviews his collaborative work with Leonore Ganschow over 20 years. Their focus has been on researching language and literacy skills learning among secondary school learners in contexts related to a foreign language curriculum. He also takes a cognitive approach, working with a range of test data and statistical analyses related to groups of individuals. His work demonstrates the need to take account of the close relationships between first and second language development across the spectrum of abilities. It also points up the interrelationship between motivation and achievement on pupils' language learning.

In Chapter 3, Carol Goldfus also takes a cognitive perspective, here to examine an intervention programme for EAL/EFL reading comprehension for adolescents with severe reading difficulties in secondary school settings. Her research approach to intervention addresses three levels of textual comprehension: word and intrasentential levels of reading skills, and a new third level, intersentential. The approach in the intervention programme offers teachers and students joint access to both the learners' difficulties and their strategies for resolving their difficulties with printed text.

In Chapter 4, Judit Kormos reviews recent literature on dyslexic language learners in contexts where students are learning English as part of the curriculum. Her review interrogates a number of cognitively oriented approaches. She argues that there is a need to move the research gaze from etic to the emic perspective, that is, from the researcher's perspective to that of the learners with dyslexia, in foreign language learning settings. She indicates a way forward for future study, which is that of drawing on sociocultural conceptualisations of learning and qualitative methodology.

In Chapter 5, Brendan Weekes and his colleagues approach dyslexia in multilingual settings from a different perspective. They are primarily interested in acquired dyslexia in bilingual adults and the intriguing question of whether language processing systems for oral reading are language specific or integrated. Their review of empirical research shows similar patterns across bilingual and monolingual speakers of different languages. They explore the question further using the explanatory potential of a theoretical computational model of oral reading, the Bilingual Interactive Activation (BIA) model.

Maria Rontou's work in Chapter 6 draws on sociocultural theory through an organisational ethnography. She analyses and interprets the implementation of national policy for inclusive provision for pedagogy and accommodation support for students with dyslexia in secondary schools in Greece. Her ethnography is informed by recent developments in activity theory to explore, through emic perspectives, the experiences of students with dyslexia and their parents, teachers and headteachers. While the study does not engage research methods for change, the ethnography shows raised awareness resulting from the study.

Jean Conteh in Chapter 7 critiques policy and practice in education systems which privilege only monolingual literacy skills for multilingual learners. Her starting point is with the growing body of research which demonstrates the cognitive and social advantages that accrue from bilingual approaches to teaching and learning. She argues that the oppressive persistence of monolingual education can be interpreted, in Vygotskian terms, as a form of cultural deprivation. Using ethnographic method and social constructivist and interpretative analytical lenses, Jean Conteh's study reveals rich multilingual literacies resources that learners can bring to classroom learning.

In Chapter 8, Bobbie Kabuto gives an account of how her daughter Emma's development of bilingual literacies proved to be integral to the development of identity and self. Three important methodological issues are illustrated. First, simultaneously developing bilingual orthographies highlights the complex, integrated relationship between them across distinct contexts. Second, we see the need for a longitudinal perspective: the collection of Emma's orthographic texts took place over four years. Third, three theoretical lenses generate the analytical frameworks to interpret Emma's emerging multilingual literacies and her construction of different identities.

Together the chapters add up to more than the sum of their parts. They provide us with a unique barometer of the state-of-the-art in thinking about dyslexia and multilingual literacy, across disciplines and research paradigms. Each chapter has been written in ways that engage us as readers and invite us to view dyslexia through different lenses, taking account of the increasing diversity of the 21st century.

Note

1   In Lindsay *et al.*'s (2006) study the measure of under- and over-representation calculated a substantial statistical difference. Pupils from a minority ethnic group are 1.5 times *more* likely than White British pupils to be identified or, conversely, are 1.5 times *less* likely to be identified with special educational need (SEN), indicating *over*-representation and *under*-representation respectively (Lindsay *et al.*, 2006: 5).

References

Artiles, A.J., Waitoller, F.R. and Neal, R. (2011) Grappling with the intersection of language and ability differences: Equity issues for Chicano/Latino students in special education. In R. Valencia (ed.) *Chicano School Failure and Success: Past, Present and Future* (3rd edn) (pp. 213–234). London: Routledge/Falmer.

Bagga-Gupta, S. (2012) Privileging identity positions and multimodal communication in textual practices: Intersectionality and the (re)negotiation of boundaries. In A. Pitkänen-Huhta and L. Holm (eds) *Literacy Practices in Transition: Perspectives from the Nordic Countries* (pp. 75–100). Bristol: Multilingual Matters.

Barton, D. and Lee, C. (2013) *Language Online: Texts and Practices on the Internet*. London: Routledge.

Blackledge, A. and Creese, A. (2009) *Multilingualism: A Critical Perspective*. London: Continuum.

British Psychological Society (1999) *Dyslexia, Literacy and Psychological Assessment* (Working Party Report). Leicester: BPS.

Cameron, D., Frazer, E., Harvey, P., Rampton, B. and Richardson, K. (1992) *Researching Language: Issues of Power and Method*. London: Routledge.

Cline, T. and Shamsi, T. (2000) *Language Needs or Special Needs? The Assessment of Learning Difficulties in Literacy Among Children Learning English as an Additional Language: A Literature Review*. London: Department for Education and Employment.

Creese, A. and Blackledge, A.J. (2010) Translanguaging in the bilingual classroom: A pedagogy for learning and teaching? *Modern Language Journal* 94 (1), 103–115.

Duchêne, A. and Heller, M. (eds) (2012) *Language in Late Capitalism: Pride and Profit*. London: Routledge.

Flewitt, R., Nind, M. and Payler, J. (2009) If she's left with books she'll just eat them: Considering inclusive multimodal literacy practices. *Journal of Early Childhood Literacy* 9 (2), 211–233.

Frith, U. (1997) Brain, mind and behaviour in dyslexia. In C. Hulme and M.J. Snowling (eds) *Dyslexia: Biology, Cognition and Intervention* (pp. 1–19). London: Whurr.

Garcia, O. (2009) *Bilingual Education in the 21st Century: A Global Perspective*. Oxford: Wiley-Blackwell.

Gillborn, D. and Youdell, D. (2000) *Rationing Education: Policy, Practice, Reform, and Equity*. Buckingham: Open University Press.

Hasson, N., Camilleri, B., Jones, C., Smith, J. and Dodd, B. (2013) Discriminating disorder from difference using dynamic assessment with bilingual children. *Child Language Teaching and Therapy* 29 (1), 57–75.

Hatcher, P., Hulme, C., Miles, J., Carroll, J., Hatcher, J., Gibbs, S., Smith, G., Bowyer-Crane,

C. and Snowling, M. (2006) Efficacy of small group reading intervention for beginning readers with reading-delay: A randomised controlled trial. *Journal of Child Psychology and Psychiatry* 47 (8), 820–827.

Heath, S.B. (1983) *Ways With Words: Language, Life, and Work in Communities and Classrooms*. Cambridge: Cambridge University Press.

Hornberger, N.H. (1989) Continua of biliteracy. *Review of Educational Research* 59 (3), 271–296.

Hornberger, N.H. and Skilton-Sylvester, E. (2000) Revisiting the continua of biliteracy: International and critical perspectives. *Language and Education* 14 (2), 96–122.

Hymes, D. (1981/1968) The ethnography of speaking. In J. Fishman (ed.) *Readings in the Sociology of Language* (pp. 99–138). The Hague: Mouton.

Kenner, C. (2000) *Home Pages*. Stoke: Trentham Books.

Kliewer, C. (1998) *Schooling Children with Down Syndrome: Toward an Understanding of Possibility*. New York: Teachers College Press.

Kress, G. and van Leeuwen, T. (2001) *Multimodal Discourse: The Modes and Media of Contemporary Communication*. London: Arnold.

Kress, G. R., Jewitt, C., Bourne, J., Franks, A., Hardcastle, J., Reid, E. and Jones, K. (2005) *English in Urban Classrooms: A Multimodal Perspective on Teaching and Learning*. London: RoutledgeFalmer.

Lacey, P., Layton, L., Miller, C., Goldbart, J. and Lawson, H. (2007) What is literacy for students with severe learning difficulties? Exploring conventional and inclusive literacy. *Journal of Research in Special Educational Needs* 7 (3), 149–160.

Li Wei (2010) Moment analysis and translanguaging space: Discursive construction of identities by multilingual Chinese youth in Britain. *Journal of Pragmatics* 43, 1222–1235.

Lindsay, G., Pather, S. and Strand, S. (2006) *Special Educational Needs and Ethnicity: Issues of Over- and Under-representation*, London: Department for Education and Skills.

Martin, D.M. (2009) *Language Disabilities in Cultural and Linguistic Diversity*. Bristol: Multilingual Matters.

Martin, D., Colesby, C. and Jhamat, K. (1997) Phonological awareness in Panjabi/English children with phonological difficulties. *Child Language Teaching and Therapy* 13 (1), 59–72.

Martin, D., Stuart-Smith, J. and Dhesi, K.K. (1998) Insiders and outsiders: Translating in a bilingual research project. In S. Hunston (ed.) *Language at Work* (pp. 109–122). Clevedon: Multilingual Matters/BAAL.

Maynard, D. and Marlaire, C. (1999) Good reasons for bad testing performance: The interactional substrate of educational testing. In D. Kovarsky, J. Duchan and M. Maxwell (eds) *Constructing (In)Competence: Disabling Evaluation of Clinical and Social Interaction* (pp. 171–196). Hillsdale, NJ: Erlbaum.

Middleton, D. and Brown, S.D. (2005) *The Social Psychology of Experience: Studies in Remembering and Forgetting*. London: Sage.

New London Group (1996) A pedagogy of multiliteracies: Designing social futures. *Harvard Educational Review* 66 (1), 60–92.

Peer, L. and Reid, G. (2000) *Multilingualism, Literacy and Dyslexia: A Challenge for Educators*. London: David Fulton.

Peña, E. and Gillam, R. (2000) Dynamic assessment of children referred for speech and language evaluations. *Dynamic Assessment: Prevailing Models and Applications* 6, 543–575.

Rassool, N. (2002) Literacy: In search of a paradigm. In J. Soler, J. Wearmouth and G. Reid (eds) *Contextualising Difficulties in Literacy Development* (pp. 17–46). London: RoutledgeFalmer, Open University, University of Edinburgh.

Rodriguez, M.V. (2005) Dominican children with special needs in New York City: Language and literacy practices. In A.C. Zentella (ed.) *Building on Strength: Language and Literacy in Latino Families and Communities* (pp. 119–133). New York: Teachers College Press/CABE.

Savage, R. (2004) Motor skills, automaticity and developmental dyslexia: A review of the research literature. *Reading and Writing* 17 (3), 301–324.

Smythe, I. (2010) *Dyslexia in the Digital Age: Making IT Work*. London: Continuum.

Stanovich, K. (1994) Annotation: Does dyslexia exist? *Journal of Child Psychology and Psychiatry* 35 (4), 579–595.

Street, B. (1984) *Literacy in Theory and Practice*. Cambridge: Cambridge University Press.

Tomasello, M. (2003) *Constructing a Language: A Usage-Based Theory of Language Acquisition*. Cambridge, MA: Harvard University Press.

Torgesen, J.K. (2005) Recent discoveries from research on remedial interventions for children with dyslexia. In M.J. Snowling and C. Hulme (eds) *The Science of Reading: A Handbook* (pp. 521–537). Malden, MA: Blackwell.

Torgesen, J.K.(2009) The response to intervention instructional model: Some outcomes from a large-scale implementation in reading first schools. *Child Development Perspectives* 3 (1), 38–40.

Trueba, H.T. (1988) English literacy acquisition: From cultural trauma to learning disabilities in minority students. *Linguistics and Education* 1, 125–151.

Van der Aa, J. and Blommaert, J. (2011) Ethnographic monitoring: Hymes' unfinished business in educational research. *Working Papers in Urban Language and Literacies. Paper* 69, 1–17.

1   Assessment Approaches for Multilingual Learners With Dyslexia

John Everatt, Gavin Reid and Gad Elbeheri

Introduction

Cross-linguistic studies of the diverse language/cultural societies in all parts of the world suggest that the manifestation of dyslexia may vary across languages. This indicates strongly a need for more dyslexia-focused research and recommendations for best practice targeted at individuals from multilingual backgrounds. One of the aims of this chapter is to review briefly current work as it relates specifically to dyslexia, in order that the reader understands some of the challenges for practice and theory in working with children learning several languages. An assumption underlying this review is that appropriate (and early) assessment procedures and tools designed to identify potential areas of difficulties and strengths are essential to practitioners, in both their initial identification of those at risk of learning difficulties and their formation of an appropriate intervention designed for the needs of the individual.

Early identification leads to more effective intervention, particularly in the areas of reading and writing (see Torgesen, 2005), and a failure to recognise difficulties can often lead to the child becoming anxious or depressed and losing self-esteem, confidence and motivation (see Elbeheri et al., 2009; Everatt & Reid, 2010; Miles, 2004). Despite the availability of screening and assessment procedures that have been developed to aid this process in, primarily, monolingual English-speaking contexts, there is a lack of work that can be used to inform best practice within a multilingual context (see Cline & Shamsi, 2000). Two of the main obstacles to this have been the lack of procedures and tools (and suitably trained testers) to assess across different language contexts, and the potential for the effects on literacy development of learning a second language to obscure the identification of dyslexia (see Cline & Reason, 1993; Peer & Reid, 2000). The following pages provide a discussion of these obstacles and the factors that may need to be considered to improve practice, based on our current research understanding.

Dyslexia in Multilingual/Multicultural Societies

One of the potential consequences of the lack of research, and a key issue that needs be raised in relation to dyslexia and multilingualism, is that the prevalence of dyslexia identified among children from dual (or multi) language backgrounds is lower than expected (based on general population samples). For example, Curnyn et al. (1991) found that bilingual learners were significantly under-represented among pupils who were assessed as having dyslexia. Similar research by Landon et al., (2000) investigated 144 Scottish primary schools and confirmed the results of the earlier Curnyn study. The Scottish research revealed that parents from ethnic minority communities are frequently excluded from involvement in the assessment process because of poor provision of interpreters (see also Diniz, 1997; Shah, 1995). The Landon et al. study also revealed a great deal of confusion among teachers about the assessment and support of bilingual learners suspected of being dyslexic. Such work has indicated that, when multilingual learners fail to make progress in the curriculum, those conducting assessments and classroom interventions should not assume that low language proficiency is necessarily the problem. There has been a trend for specialist teachers and psychologists to misdiagnose or ignore dyslexia indicators in multilingual students because of the multiplicity of possible causes for failure to make progress and the risk of a 'false positive' result (see discussions in Peer & Reid, 2000). Lack of suitable test materials, cultural perceptions of dyslexia, policies for identification and classroom practices all affect the nature of the support for bilingual learners suspected of being, or diagnosed as being, dyslexic.

Berryman and Wearmouth (2009) argue that dyslexia is commonly understood as an explanation of difficulties in literacy from a cognitive perspective (i.e. as a set of factors within the brain/individual). This level of explanation, they argue, ignores the impact of culture. They suggest that research shows the benefits to literacy learning that accrue when schools work to address the cultural backgrounds of the children they are teaching. Such views are supported by theorists such as McNaughton (1995) who discuss socialisation values that match home culture. This is relevant across the modern world, as virtually every country has individuals who derive from a range of different cultural backgrounds. Dyslexia, therefore, should be seen from a broader, more culturally aware perspective. Both assessment and intervention practices need to take account of these potential differences (see also Mcfarlane et al., 2000).

In a report by a working party of the Division of Educational and Child Psychology of the British Psychological Society (BPS) on Dyslexia,

Literacy and Psychological Assessment (BPS, 1999), it was argued that an emphasis must be placed on culture-fair assessment, and that indicators such as phonological difficulties and letter-naming speed in the language of tuition should be the focus of a diagnosis. Although culture-fair assessment is crucial (Cline, 1998), analysis of test performance within specific cultural and linguistic groups can itself also help to identify those items which consistently lead to cultural confusion or misperception. Usmani (2000) suggests that the bilingual/bicultural child may have a broad range of thinking skills that can go undetected if the professional is unaware of associated cultural values or fails to understand them in relation to the assessment. Usmani further suggests that the 'big dip' in the performance of some bilingual children noted in later primary education may be explained by a failure of professionals to understand and appreciate these cultural values and the actual level of competence of the bilingual child in relation to conceptual development and competence in thinking skills. As suggested by Palincsar and Brown (1984), better thinking skills should lead to improved comprehension in readers who are struggling with acquiring literacy.

Although assessments need to be culturally appropriate, another reason for the under-representation of dyslexia in multilingual groups may be the view that such learners have processing difficulties that are due to poor language proficiency rather than an educationally based learning difficulty, such as dyslexia (see Dal, 2008). Hence, appropriate assessments need to take into account any language factors that may be related to alternative causes of reading problems.

Language, Phonology and Orthography

Well designed assessment procedures are particularly important where an observed behavioural problem may be due to a number of underlying reasons, and optimal effective intervention may depend on distinguishing between them. A problem with learning to read English could be due to an underlying English-language processing deficit (e.g. a phonological weakness – the dominant causal viewpoint in research on dyslexia: see Snowling, 2000), poor educational experience (e.g. lack of appropriate schooling) or incomplete acquisition of English as a second language (the individual may be new to learning the English language). Each of these may require specific interventions, such as a phonologically based intervention, an increase in school experience or greater language experience. Although good educational practice (pedagogy) should support learning in all cases, an intensive phonological intervention that supports literacy acquisition among dyslexic students may be inappropriate for English-language learners who have appropriately developed phonological awareness skills.

In most cases, an assessment procedure targeted at identifying literacy learning difficulties would include determination of the child's (or adult's) language skills, given that the written form is used to represent language and those with weak language would be expected to struggle with literacy learning. If the individual has difficulty understanding language, then comprehending or producing meaningful written text may also suffer. In addition, phonological skills have been considered to support the translation of writing into a form that can be used by already developed language processes. Such phonological skills refer to those used to process basic sounds within the language, that is, to recognise that /dog/ begins with a /d/ sound. There is a large body of research that is consistent with phonological processing skills being a vital component in effective literacy learning and with a phonological deficit being related to the literacy problems faced by children with dyslexia (e.g. Gillon, 2004; Snowling, 2000; Stanovich, 1988). Poor scores on measures of phonological processing are good predictors of early problems with literacy learning (e.g. Puolakanaho *et al.*, 2008) and are associated with literacy weaknesses, and dyslexia, throughout development and into adulthood (Beaton *et al.*, 1997).

Data relating literacy difficulties to phonological deficits have mainly been derived from studies of English-speaking individuals. However, relationships between phonological skills and literacy learning have been found across a number of languages (e.g. Smythe *et al.*, 2008; Ziegler *et al.*, 2010). Despite this, there is still a need for a phonological deficit to be confirmed as the main factor that can be used to identify dyslexia across different orthographies (see discussions in Smythe *et al.*, 2004). One of the reasons for caution here is that children learning a script (an orthography in the present context) with a more consistent relationship between written symbols (letters/graphemes) and language sounds (phonemes) than that found in English seem to show faster progress in literacy, and process language at the level of the phoneme earlier, than those learning a less regular orthography, such as English (see Goswami, 2000; Seymour *et al.*, 2003).

The view that English is less transparent (i.e. the relation between written form and language sounds is less clear in English) than most other orthographies has led some to question the universality of current theories about literacy learning. Basically, the argument is that most theories about literacy have been derived from research on English, which is an atypical orthography in that most other orthographies are more transparent than English (see discussions in Share, 2008). Therefore, research is needed on more typical orthographies to confirm the findings derived from research on English before we can consider them generalisable to other languages.

Additionally, compared with children learning English literacy skills, phonological awareness deficits may create fewer problems when learning a regular orthography since the simple rules or correspondences between letters and sounds will be less tasking of a weak phonological system. That is, even if a phonological deficit does lead to literacy learning problems, these may be less severe when learning a more transparent orthography. As such, the transparency of the script is a factor that may lead to variations between languages in the ease of literacy acquisition, the manifestation of literacy deficits and the appropriateness of particular assessment procedures. For example, whereas assessments of accuracy in word reading tasks seem appropriate to assess literacy skills in English, such tools may be less effective in more transparent orthographies, where, instead, literacy assessment procedures might more appropriately focus on measuring fluency, or speed, of processing (see Smythe et al., 2004). Determining the speed at which a child can produce a certain level of accuracy (fluency of performance) has been found to identify those children who may be able to achieve reasonable levels of accuracy, but whose slow speeds are indicative of finding word processing effortful. These children may struggle in literacy classes and when text understanding or production is required, and also may show poor acquisition of literacy-related language skills (see also Everatt et al., 2010).

Dyslexia and Biliteracy

Research on children learning to read and write in two orthographies has confirmed some of these concerns regarding orthographic transparency. For example, in research on bilingual children in the Philippines and Namibia, Everatt et al. (2010) found that word reading and non-word decoding developed at different rates for Filipino versus English and for Herero versus English, respectively. Both Filipino and Herero have relatively simple relationships between graphemes and phonemes, making it fairly easy to learn conversion rules for decoding. As might be expected, these more transparent orthographies showed good learning rates for word decoding and, hence, most of the bilingual children studied acquired good levels of accuracy in word-level literacy tasks in Filipino or Herero. Yet, despite these clear differences in acquisition, phonological skills were still the main predictor of a child's literacy learning in both languages. These findings suggest that literacy learning is dependent on phonological skills irrespective of orthographic transparency. Indeed, in the Filipino/English data, equivalent amounts of the variability in reading among the grade 1 children tested could be predicted by phonological processing measures of decoding, phonological awareness, rapid naming and auditory short-term memory. Furthermore, research by Everatt et al. (2002) has suggested that the assessment of underlying phonological skills affords the potential to distinguish individuals with dyslexia from those who are reading in an additional language, despite equally poor literacy skills being presented by both groups. Therefore, assessments of phonological skills may be a useful tool to identify dyslexia in many language/literacy contexts.

These findings may be interpreted as meaning that an assessment in English can replace an assessment in the other language of the bilingual learner, since the English assessment measures are highly predictive of skills in the other language. However, again, these conclusions need to be treated with caution. Data from the Filipino/English work suggest that measures of Filipino phonological awareness were better at identifying those with poor English literacy skills than tests of English phonological awareness skills. When Filipino and English measures were combined in a bilingual assessment, profiles of difficulties better mirrored profiles typically found with assessments of monolingual English children; that is, there was evidence of deficits in most areas of phonological processing (see Everatt *et al.*, 2010).

Hence, there seems to be a complex relationship between phonologically based language skills and literacy learning. This may not be surprising given the evidence for a reciprocal relationship between language and literacy (Perfetti *et al.*, 1987). The development of phonemic awareness (i.e. recognising sounds at the level of the phoneme) comes with increased linguistic experience and formal reading instruction. Awareness of sounds at the level of the phoneme seems to be a consequence of literacy learning as much as it is a predictor of future literacy levels. Such a relationship may well cross languages in bilingual and/or second language development and go beyond phonologically based language skills. The Filipino/English bilingual data show how phonologically based language skills can be a good predictor of literacy in another language. Similarly, in the Herero/English data, second (English) language measures of phonological awareness predicted more variability in both first (Herero) and second (English) language literacy than first (Herero) language phonological awareness measures. In a longitudinal study by Sparks *et al.* (2009), language 1 literacy skills in elementary school predicted language 2 language levels in later schooling and adulthood, consistent with literacy skills in one language influencing language competence in another.

Greater exposure to print can lead to improvements in vocabulary, general knowledge and other skills assessed in commonly used language tests. Vocabulary size may be increased by literacy experience because rare words are more likely to be encountered in print than in oral language (Nagy & Anderson, 1984). With increased reading, an individual's general knowledge also should improve, leading to better performance in verbal ability tests. The average person will encounter more complex syntactic structures in print than they would in speech, which again should lead to improved development of language skills. Exposure to different forms of language (including the written form) may also serve to increase meta-linguistic skills (see Koda, 2007), that is, to increase the individual's ability to understand language in a non-language-specific sense.

Such cross-language effects will, most likely, interact with environmental (educational) factors experienced by the child. Learning the relationship between letters and sounds in a more transparent orthography may make decoding processes sufficiently well practised for them to support literacy learning even when it is less effective in a lower-transparency second orthography. In the context studied in the Philippines, where sound–symbol relationships were explicitly taught as part of literacy learning, there were relatively few children with poor English-language decoding skills. In contrast, the Namibian school system did not focus on the relationship between graphemes and phonemes, even when learning Herero, and many children showed poor levels of English word reading and spelling. Under the right circumstances, learning of a second language may strengthen cognitive processing, and cross-linguistic transfer of phonological processing skills may mean that phonological knowledge of two sound systems will facilitate the development of first and second languages (see Bialystok *et al.*, 2005).

However, learning a second language will not produce only positive outcomes. Errors can be caused by an overextension of an analogy learnt in a first language but applied incorrectly in the second – and the more similar the two orthographies, the greater the potential for these over-generalisations to occur. Indeed, both the potential positive and negative consequences of learning a second language may depend on relationships/commonalities between the two languages/orthographies learnt (see Bialystok *et al.*, 2005). Additionally, some learners of English as a second language may struggle to understand relatively uncommon words in the second language that may be fairly familiar to their monolingual English peers – and weak vocabulary can be a barrier to comprehension. Dal (2008) has argued that bilingual students can exhibit an auditory–verbal processing delay which means that they take longer to develop fluency in language-related processes. This, in addition to cultural differences and unfamiliar vocabulary, can result in an assumption that difficulties are due to bilingualism when in fact the child is demonstrating dyslexic difficulties. Furthermore, Dal has suggested that the underlying problems in language processing experienced by many dyslexic students can make learning any new language difficult. If this is the case, the development of language skills will be delayed specifically among dyslexic individuals, potentially further negating any benefits from early identification. Again, the reciprocal relationship between these factors can increase problems in identification. Further research targeted at specifying these relationships, therefore, is vital to inform best practice in dyslexia assessment.

As argued above, skills in one language may support relative weaknesses in a second and such cross-language skills transfer has been found in quite distinct languages/orthographies, such as Arabic and English. In ongoing research investigating the writing skills of Arabic adolescents learning English as a second language, text coherence as a measure of the production of meaningful English text showed small correlations with English vocabulary levels, but larger relationships with syntactic awareness; and the latter effect was larger than would be expected based on data from monolingual English students. This may be because such syntactic awareness skills are highly useful in producing the appropriate written form of Arabic and their use has transferred to English writing tasks. Hence, skills learnt in one language/orthography may transfer and support development in the other language/orthography, and a weakness in one area may be supported by skills in another. Therefore, specific features of (including problems with) literacy learning that we observe in an assessment of a bilingual/second language learner may be as much a result of cross-language skills transfer as a feature the literacy learning *per se*. Assessment procedures that are sensitive to such influences should lead to better conclusions.

Overall, despite differences across languages/orthographies, the majority of the evidence discussed supports the view that phonological deficits are an underlying cause of literacy learning problems across languages and bilingual populations. However, word-level literacy acquisition has been shown to be faster when learning a more transparent orthography (given commonality of other relevant factors, such as appropriate learning opportunity) and the manifestation of difficulties in literacy learning can vary with the orthography learnt. The evidence argues also for a reciprocal relationship between literacy development and language skills, particularly with respect to phonological processing, but also with other aspects of language, such as vocabulary, syntactic awareness and metalinguistic skills. These interrelationships show evidence of cross-language/orthography transfer, which can lead to positive outcomes when skills learnt in one language support development in a second, but can also produce errors, for example if over-generalisations of rules across languages occur. Hence, bilingualism, or second language learning, need not be a barrier to literacy acquisition, but the features of literacy learning (and language skills) presented may show influences of the languages used by the child. This has important implications for assessment procedures. This is not to argue that assessment practices should stop while bilingual procedures are developed: the evidence still indicates that assessments in one language can be informative of difficulties in another. Rather, recognition of the potential effects of cross-language influences may help explain the child's performance in both language and literacy tests. As research and practice in this field increases, our understanding of these interrelationships/influences should improve, leading to more informed assessments.

English, Arabic and Other Languages

English has been the focus of much second language research. However, as discussed above, research in other languages needs to be considered. Arabic is an interesting language to study since, like English, it is used as an additional language/orthography by a large number of individuals from varied home language backgrounds: it is the language of the Koran and, therefore, Arabic text needs to be learnt to the level of pronunciation by all Muslims. Additionally, the form of Arabic used in written text is not the same as that spoken in everyday conversation by Arab children; a child will learn to speak one of the many dialects of Arabic spoken within a local context (a particular country or region within a country). The written form, however, is based on a standard form of Arabic used across the Arab world and may vary from the child's spoken form in terms of vocabulary, morpho-syntactic rules and even phonological forms. The common form (Modern Standard Arabic or MSA), typically, is learnt during formal schooling and as part of the process of learning to read and write. This difference between the local spoken form and the standard form used for specific purposes of general communication and in Arabic writing (referred to as diglossia) has led some to argue that all Arab children have to acquire a second language in learning to read and write. Similar to some of the bilingual contexts discussed above, confusions between the different sound forms in the local dialect versus MSA have been found (see Saiegh-Haddad, 2005). Indeed, these differences have led Saiegh-Haddad (2005) to argue that phonological processing strategies may not support Arabic literacy acquisition as well as in other orthographies. Although it is the case that measures of phonological processing are predictive of reading levels among Arab children, and poor Arabic readers show weak phonological decoding and low levels of phonological awareness in comparison with matched normal readers (see Elbeheri & Everatt, 2007), the level of prediction of Arabic literacy provided by phonological processing skills has been less than expected from research in other languages (Elbeheri et al., 2006; Saiegh-Haddad, 2005).

Therefore, more accurate assessment may be provided by the inclusion of measures of other processing skills. For example, work to develop Arabic language assessment measures by Elbeheri and colleagues has focused on phonological skills and reading and writing ability, but has also included measures of orthographic and morphology processing (see Elbeheri et al., 2011; Mahfoudhi et al., 2010), as well as working memory, in order to take account of the specific features of the language/orthography in which the assessment is taking place. Similar test development work has been conducted in other languages (see Smythe et al., 2004). It may be that further such work will provide assessment tools across a range of languages that can be used to support assessment practices in a multilingual setting.

Assessment Practices

Although there are a number of screening and diagnostic tests used to assess dyslexic children, most have been developed for use with monolingual, usually Western-cultural populations, which may account, to a large extent, for the underestimation or misdiagnosis of dyslexia in bilingual children – and for the reluctance of practitioners to use such measures before language experience has reached a certain level (see Reid, 2009). Assessment procedures that have been developed specifically for the bilingual learner tend to focus on checklists, or questionnaires/interviews, or to use diagnostic measures that have been translated from English-language equivalents (though see the end of the previous section of this chapter for examples of assessment measures developed for different languages/orthographies). It is important, however, as it is in all cases of dyslexia, to treat the bilingual dyslexic child as an individual and, therefore, screening and diagnostic data need to be adapted and interpreted accordingly.

Many of the measures used in screening procedures can be used in full diagnostic assessments and, therefore, screening can be seen as the first step towards diagnosis. However, this level of assessment can be regarded as incomplete, and further information about skills and learning may be vital in determining strengths and difficulties, as well as to inform support and intervention (see also Everatt et al., 2008). Additional information, typically, will be gained via standardised skills/curriculum assessments. However, it needs to be recognised that a full assessment is a process, and that process may well need to consider the student in different types of learning contexts, for instance determining whether problems encountered under test conditions with strangers are also evident in reports from parents and teachers. In a study by Reid et al. (2005) of all education authorities in Scotland, the researchers found that 36 different tests or assessment procedures were used, but that none of these formal procedures were designed for children with a first language other than English. It is important, therefore, that if such standardised diagnostic tests are used, they are supplemented by observation criteria which can incorporate the child's performance across curricular areas as well as in different learning contexts.

In view of the need to avoid cultural bias in assessment it is important to consider alternative forms of assessment, such as 'dynamic assessment'. The goal of dynamic assessment is to evaluate learning ability and to gain information useful for more effective instruction. This approach essentially links assessment and teaching and highlights the child's learning process. Focusing on dynamic rather than static assessment, particularly among bilingual children (Reid, 2009; Usmani, 2000), has the potential to take into account elements of the test situation, such as language skills, and links with teaching in scaffolding and building language concepts.

Assessment of learning style may also be a useful alternative form of assessment in order to consider the bilingual child as an individual learner. There is evidence that learning style, both environmental and cognitive, can affect educational progress, particularly in literacy (Milgram et al., 1993; Mortimore, 2007; Reid & Stradova, 2008), and may be useful when developing an assessment protocol for students with dyslexia. Additionally, Dunn and Milgram (1993) examined the learning styles of students from different cultures and noted the diversity of these styles both within and across cultures. Hence, cultural background may need to be taken into account when basing conclusions on such assessments.

The point here is that these alternative assessment protocols underline the view that assessment is much more than testing (Reid, 2009). Assessment may be better seen as part of the process of information gathering and mutual learning from parents, teachers and other professionals. This process, therefore, will take place over time and consider the learning environment as well as linguistic and cultural differences between the individuals involved in the process.

It can be argued that the nature and process of assessment procedures and tests for multilingual students will differ from those used for other children. It is important, therefore, to develop a framework for guidelines for assessment, as well as for intervention. This should include background information on the student, assessment of the classroom environment and school culture, classroom observations over time, curriculum-based assessment, the use of appropriate formal standardised tests and the monitoring of teaching approaches. It is important that the views of parents are considered as well as cultural factors and cultural norms.

Classroom Practices/Interventions

Research indicates that the acquisition of written language skills is supported by an awareness of the sound system (see discussion above). Not surprisingly, therefore, training in phonological awareness has turned out to be one of the most powerful components of successful intervention programmes for students at risk of dyslexia. By extension, therefore, an important goal of teaching a second language to dyslexic students is to help them become aware of this sound system and its relationship to the written form. A well developed phonological awareness system will enhance dyslexic students' skills in both word reading and spelling in the foreign language as well as their pronunciation of new vocabulary (see for example D'Angiulli et al., 2005; Lipa & Siegel, 2007).

Phonological awareness can be improved by integrating games into classroom practice, such as rhyming games, and tasks that involve subtracting and changing sounds within spoken words (change the /p/ sound in 'pig' to a /b/ sound and what do you get?). Two important points here are that: (1) for interventions to improve literacy acquisition, the link with reading and writing needs to be made clear for the child with a learning difficulty; and (2) for the learner with phonological processing problems, as is the case with dyslexic learners, more time and training may be needed to reach an acceptable level of skill. In the USA, the National Reading Panel's report (National Institute of Child Health and Human Development, 2000) of a meta-analysis conducted on the efficacy of interventions concluded that: (1) instruction based on phonological awareness works significantly better than other forms of instruction for improving spelling, reading accuracy and comprehension; (2) when used with accompanying letters, phonological awareness helps typically developing and at-risk children develop their phonemic awareness better than training in phonological awareness without manipulation of letters; and (3) when incorporated in programmes of 5–18 hours, training in phonological awareness results in better progress than when it is taught in programmes of shorter or longer duration. The report also suggests that phonological awareness programmes are effective when taught by either teacher or computer but best results in terms of transfer to reading occur when training is coupled with manipulating letters, the focus is on segmenting and blending, and the instructional group size is small.

Phonologically based interventions that link to literacy, therefore, seem to provide a basis on which to support literacy learning across a range of children within different learning contexts, including those from a bi- or multilingual background. However, it is important that the child's strengths (including competence in languages other than English and cultural experience), motivation and self-esteem, and learning styles are included in the development of classroom programmes. As teaching approaches are selected and devised, through collaboration between the class or subject teacher and learning support staff, it is important to ensure that, as far as possible, these approaches are incorporated into the child's daily curricular activities rather than as separate programmes of work. The more they are integrated into normal learning activities, the more likely they are to influence those activities.

However, it is important also to recognise the specific skills that may be needed to support bilingual students. For example, Landon *et al.* (2000) have noted that the difficulties many bilingual learners have with articulating, especially, English vowels and final consonantal morphemes may impede recognition and production of these sounds. Furthermore, speakers of syllable-timed languages (e.g. Cantonese) may have difficulty in hearing unstressed syllables in stress-timed English utterances. Previous experience of reading a more logographically based script, as opposed to an alphabetic one, may also cause difficulties with analogical reading for a literate Chinese pupil (Goswami & Bryant, 1990; McBride-Chang *et al.*, 2004). Therefore, more practice in recognising rhyme and syllable (or other units of the language) may be necessary for learners from certain language backgrounds.

The repetition of information/concepts that have been learnt poorly will be required with many children with learning difficulties, and this will be true also for those with dyslexia from a bi- or multilingual background. Repetition leads to increased practice, which is often necessary for children struggling with learning. Multisensory learning methods also can be useful to reinforce ideas, by presenting information in different ways so as to avoid the boredom produced by simple repetition. Multisensory strategies have the defining characteristic of presenting information in different forms so that the child can see, hear and even feel the ideas presented, in addition to the child producing them by tracing, drawing, writing and speaking.

Presenting information in these different ways may also make it easier for the child to remember the information, by reinforcing the information in a way that the child finds accessible and fun (an amusing image can often be recalled to mind more easily than a neutral word). The fact that language need not be the primary medium of learning also is likely to be advantageous to bi- and multilingual learners. It is vital for information to be presented to the dyslexic learner on different occasions and in different ways to help the information pass from short-term to long-term memory, thus ensuring automaticity. Spelling, for example, can be taught initially in a multisensory way, leading to over-learning through the use of games, computer activities and word webs. Learning and over-learning will be most effective for monolingual and bilingual learners when words are presented and used in meaningful contexts, and when the need to use the word derives from the pupil and not from the teacher. For bilingual learners this clearly has implications for the creation of culturally sensitive learning environments and tasks.

It must be remembered that a dyslexic learner who successfully spells a word during a spelling test will not necessarily spell the same word correctly in a piece of imaginative writing, until automaticity has been achieved. This is because the child's full concentration is on the spelling alone in the first case, but is focused on creating a story in the second. While correct spelling is becoming automatic, critical proofreading is a skill which must be taught. The child, freed from the main task of creating a story, is then likely to self-correct many spelling errors.

Process writing, that is, collaborative drafting and redrafting of written text in multilingual groups, has been found to be a useful approach for bilingual learners in developing compositional and editing skills (Brown & Campione, 1994; Dunn & Milgram, 1993). Such compositional and editing skills have been related to the ability to monitor performance, which is often considered from the perspective of metacognitive awareness, and there is a view that children with dyslexia may have poor metacognitive awareness, particularly in relation to print and literacy (Tunmer & Chapman, 1996). When children are learning to read words, they develop 'recognition', then 'understanding' and then 'transferable' skills, which means that they need to develop concepts and an understanding of the text before they can use the new word or text in other contexts; this transferring of skills is crucial to the development of metacognitive awareness. To achieve metacognitive awareness, children usually develop schemata (children's specific understanding, from their perspective, of a situation or text). To achieve schemata of a situation, children need to be able to express their understanding of the situation verbally or in written form, and to identify the specific concepts and how these relate to the overall picture. The teacher, through a process called scaffolding, helps to build up this understanding and the conceptual and schematic development of the child. Reid (2007) suggests that such metacognitive approaches are essential to provide readers with the independent skills needed for full engagement in the reading process and this is more crucial for learners with dyslexia, particularly those who are bilingual. Metacognitive strategies consist of advance organising (e.g. skimming and previewing the text), selecting a purpose for reading and scanning to achieve that purpose, as well as self-monitoring and editing, and reviewing the effectiveness of the completed task and the learning experience. Classroom approaches for dyslexic students with more than one language need to look beyond the linguistic features, to take account of the student's complete learning profile. Intervention should be individualised and comprehensive.

Concluding Comments

One of the key challenges facing educators in relation to bilingualism and dyslexia is that of identification. In order to address this, it is important to develop assessment materials in the language being taught, but to make those materials culture-fair. Additionally, it may be necessary to develop assessment materials in the first language of the child to assess whether dyslexia is present and affecting the development of skills in literacy in that first language. Overall, the majority of the evidence discussed supports the view that phonological deficits are an underlying cause of problems in literacy learning across languages and among bilingual populations, and that training in these skills can support literacy development within populations learning English as either a first or a second language, particularly when the link to reading and writing is made explicit. The evidence also suggests that bi- or multilingualism, or second language learning, need not be a barrier to literacy acquisition, but recognition of the potential effects of cross-language influences may help explain the child's performance in language-related assessments. Hence, further research in different languages/orthographies is needed to identify of the main features of a language/orthography that influence performance in language/literacy tasks, and to indicate how these features may interact in bilingual/second language contexts. Through such practitioner-focused research, better assessment measures should be developed and assessment procedures should be more likely to determine the reason for the level/type of performance shown by a child/adult, including those within a bi- or multilingual context.

The evidence from the research so far argues that assessments of children learning more than one language should include appropriate standardised measurements of literacy skills in the language of education (which in many second language contexts is English). This would include measures of word reading accuracy, but assessments of fluency and comprehension should also be considered with bilingual children. Assessment of the level of a range of phonological processing skills acquired in the second language should also be included; awareness, speed of access and retention are all potentially informative of problems experienced by the individual. However, phono-logically based assessments in the individual's first language would be useful to support any conclusions drawn about the learning of the second language. In addition, more general cognitive measures should be considered, to assess the general level of functioning. These may be important to inform areas of weakness and strength (for example, non-verbal ability can compensate for problems with language, and may be an area of relative strength for the dyslexic individual that can support learning). However, care is needed to avoid cultural biases in these more general skills areas, which are often associated with IQ. Finally, a determination of language skills in the second language would be advisable, although first language measures also would support decisions about comorbid problems (such as specific language im-pairments).

As discussed in this chapter, these more formal assessments and standardised tools can be supported by alternative assessment procedures, such as dynamic assessment or a consideration of learning styles. Working with parents and first language teachers should also be considered, to give background details on learning/functioning. These can then feed into recom-mendations for teaching/intervention. Currently, the evidence suggests that similar procedures used to support learning in first language children can be useful in supporting second language learners; phonological awareness interventions linked to word decoding strategies can be particularly useful, but so can wider curriculum strategies, such as multisensory learning, as these can facilitate repetition and support memorisation and metacognitive awareness, which in turn help with understanding, learning and independ-ence. However, the specific features that the bi- or multilingual child brings to the educational environment mean that further research should focus on children identified as dyslexic and who are learning to read and write in an additional language.

References

Beaton, A., McDougall, S. and Singleton, C. (eds) (1997) Special issue: Dyslexia in literate adults. *Journal of Research in Reading* 20 (1).
Berryman, M. and Wearmouth, J. (2009) Responsive approaches to literacy learning within cultural contexts. In G. Reid (ed.) *The Routledge Companion to Dyslexia* (pp. 337–353). London: Routledge.
Bialystok, E., McBride-Chang, C. and Luk, G. (2005) Bilingualism, language proficiency, and learning to read in two writing systems. *Journal of Educational Psychology* 97, 580–590.
BPS (1999) *Dyslexia, Literacy and Psychological Assessment. Report of a Working Party of the Division of Educational and Child Psychology of the British Psychological Society.* Leicester: British Psychological Society.
Brown, A.L. and Campione, J.C. (1994) Guided discovery in a community of learners. In K. McGilly (ed.) *Classroom Lessons: Integrating Cognitive Theory and Classroom Practice* (pp. 229–270). Cambridge, MA: MIT Press.

Cline, T. (1998) The assessment of special educational needs for bilingual children. *British Journal of Special Education* 25, 159–163.

Cline, T. and Reason, R. (1993) Specific reading difficulties (dyslexia): Equal opportunities issues. *British Journal of Special Education* 20, 30–34.

Cline T. and Shamsi T. (2000) *Language Needs or Special Needs? The Assessment of Learning Difficulties in Literacy Among Children Learning English as an Additional Language: A Literature Review.* London: Department for Education and Employment.

Curnyn, J., Wallace, I., Kistan, S. and McLaren, M. (1991) *Special Educational Needs and Ethnic Minority Pupils.* Glasgow: Strathclyde Education Department.

Dal, M. (2008) Dyslexia and foreign language learning. In G. Reid, A. Fawcett, F. Manis and L. Siegel (eds) *Sage Dyslexia Handbook* (pp. 439–454). London: Sage.

D'Angiulli, A., Siegel, L.S. and Maggi, S. (2005) Literacy instruction, SES, and word-reading achievement in English-language learners and children with English as a first language: A longitudinal study. *Learning Disabilities Research and Practice* 19, 202–213.

Diniz, F.A. (1997) Working with families in a multi-ethnic European context. In B. Carpenter (ed.) *Families in Context: Emerging Trends in Family Support* (pp. 107–120). London: David Fulton Publishers.

Dunn, R. and Milgram, R.M. (1993) Learning styles of gifted students in diverse cultures. In R.M. Milgram, R. Dunn and G.E. Price (eds) *Teaching and Counseling Gifted and Talented Adolescents: An International Learning Style Perspective* (pp. 3–23). Westport, CT: Praeger.

Elbeheri, G. and Everatt, J. (2007) Literacy ability and phonological processing skills amongst dyslexic and non-dyslexic speakers of Arabic. *Reading and Writing* 20, 273–294.

Elbeheri, G., Everatt, J., Reid, G. and Al-Mannai, H. (2006) Dyslexia assessment in Arabic. *Journal of Research in Special Educational Needs* 6, 143–152.

Elbeheri, G., Everatt, J. and Al-Malki, M. (2009) The incidence of dyslexia among young offenders in Kuwait. *Dyslexia* 15, 86–104.

Elbeheri, G., Everatt, J., Mahfoudhi, A., Al-Diyar, M.A. and Taibah, N. (2011) Orthographic processing and reading comprehension among Arabic speaking mainstream and LD children. *Dyslexia* 17, 123–142.

Everatt, J. and Reid, G. (2010) Motivating children with dyslexia. In J. Fletcher, F. Parkhill and G. Gillon (eds) *Motivating Literacy Learners in Today's World* (pp. 67–78). Wellington: NZCER Press.

Everatt, J., Smythe, I., Ocampo, D. and Veii, K. (2002) Dyslexia assessment of the bi-scriptal reader. *Topics in Language Disorders* 22, 32–45.

Everatt J., Weeks, S. and Brooks, P. (2008) Profiles of strengths and weaknesses in dyslexia and other learning difficulties. *Dyslexia* 14, 16–41.

Everatt J., Ocampo D., Veii, K., Nenopoulou, S., Smythe I., Al-Mannai, H. and Elbeheri, G. (2010) Dyslexia in biscriptal readers. In N. Brunswick, S. McDougall and P. de Mornay Davies (eds) *Reading and Dyslexia in Different Orthographies* (pp. 221–245). Hove: Psychology Press.

Gillon, G.T. (2004) *Phonological Awareness: From Research to Practice.* New York: Guilford Press.

Goswami, U. (2000) Phonological representations, reading development and dyslexia: Towards a cross-linguistic theoretical framework. *Dyslexia* 6, 133–151.

Goswami, U. and Bryant, P. (1990) *Phonological Skills and Learning to Read.* Hove: Psychology Press.

Koda, K. (2007) Reading and language learning: Cross-linguistic constraints on second language reading development. *Language Learning* 57, 1–44.

Landon, J., Reid, G. and Deponio, P. (2000) Dyslexia and bilingualism: Implications for assessment, teaching and learning. In L. Peer and G. Reid (eds) *Multilingualism, Literacy and Dyslexia: A Challenge for Educators.* London: David Fulton Publishers.

Lipa, O. and Siegel, L.S. (2007) The development of reading skills in children with English as a second language. *Scientific Studies of Reading* 11, 105–131.

Mahfoudhi, A., Elbeheri, G., Al-Rashidi, M. and Everatt, J. (2010) The role of morphological awareness in reading comprehension among typical and learning disabled native Arabic speakers. *Journal of Learning Disabilities* 43, 500–514.

McBride-Chang, C., Bialystok, E., Chong, K.K.Y. and Li, Y. (2004) Levels of phonological awareness in three cultures. *Journal of Experimental Child Psychology* 89, 93–111.

Mcfarlane, A., Glynn, T., Presland, I. and Greening, S. (2000) Maori culture and literacy learning: Bicultural approaches. In L. Peer and G. Reid (eds) *Multilingualism, Literacy and Dyslexia: A Challenge for Educators* (pp. 120–128). London: David Fulton Publishers.

McNaughton, S. (1995) *Patterns of Emerging Literacy: Processes of Development and Transition.* Auckland: Oxford University Press.

Miles, T.R. (ed.) (2004) *Dyslexia and Stress* (2nd edn). London: Whurr.

Milgram, R.M., Dunn, R. and Price, G.E. (eds) (1993) *Teaching and Counseling Gifted and Talented Adolescents: An International Learning Style Perspective.* Westport, CT: Praeger Publishers.

Mortimore, T. (2007) *Dyslexia and Learning Styles: A Practitioners' Handbook.* London: Wiley.

Nagy, W. and Anderson, R. (1984) How many words are there in printed school English? *Reading Research Quarterly* 19, 304–330.

National Institute of Child Health and Human Development (2000) *Report of the National Reading Panel. Teaching Children to Read: An Evidence-Based Assessment of the Scientific Research Literature on Reading and Its Implications for Instruction.* Washington, DC: US Government Printing Office.

Palincsar, A. and Brown, A. (1984) Reciprocal teaching of comprehension fostering and comprehension monitoring activities. *Cognition and Instruction* 1, 117–175.

Peer, L. and Reid, G. (eds) (2000) *Multilingualism, Literacy and Dyslexia.* London: David Fulton Publishers.

Perfetti, C.A., Beck, I., Bell, L.C. and Hughes, C. (1987) Phonemic knowledge and learning to read are reciprocal: A longitudinal study of first grade children. *Merrill-Palmer Quarterly* 33, 283–319.

Puolakanaho, A., Ahonen, T., Aro, M., Eklund, K., Leppanen, P.H.T., Poikkeus, A-M., Tolvanen, A., Torppa, M. and Lyytinen, H. (2008) Developmental links of very early phonological and language skills to second grade reading outcomes. *Journal of Learning Disabilities* 41, 353–370.

Reid, G. (2007) *Learning Styles and Inclusion.* London: Sage Publications.

Reid, G. (2009) *Dyslexia: A Practitioners' Handbook* (4th edn). Chichester: Wiley.

Reid, G. and Stradova, I. (2008) Dyslexia and learning styles: Overcoming the barriers to learning. In G. Reid, A. Fawcett, F. Manis and L. Siegel (eds) *Sage Dyslexia Handbook* (pp. 369–380). London: Sage Publications.

Reid, G., Deponio, P. and Petch, L.D. (2005) Identification, assessment and intervention: Implications of an audit of dyslexia policy and practice in Scotland. *Dyslexia* 11, 203–216.

Saiegh-Haddad, E. (2005) Correlates of reading fluency in Arabic: Diglossic and ortho-graphic factors. *Reading and Writing* 18, 559–582.

Seymour, P.H.K., Aro, M. and Erskine, J.M. (2003) Foundation literacy acquisition in European orthographies. *British Journal of Psychology* 94, 143–174.

Shah, R. (1995) *The Silent Minority: Children with Disabilities in Asian Families* (revised edn). London: National Children's Bureau.

Share, D.L. (2008) On the Anglocentricities of current reading research and practice: The perils of overreliance on an 'outlier' orthography. *Psychological Bulletin* 134, 584–615.

Smythe, I., Everatt, J. and Salter, R. (eds) (2004) *The International Book of Dyslexia.* London: Wiley.

Smythe, I., Everatt, J., Al-Menaye, N., He, X., Capellini, S., Gyarmathy, E. and Siegel, L. (2008) Predictors of word level literacy amongst grade 3 children in five diverse languages. *Dyslexia* 14, 170–187.

Snowling, M.J. (2000) *Dyslexia* (2nd edn). Oxford: Blackwell.

Sparks, R., Patton, J., Ganschow, L. and Humbach, N. (2009) Long-term cross linguistic transfer of skills from L1 to L2. *Language Learning* 59, 203–243.

Stanovich, K.E. (1988) Explaining the differences between the dyslexic and the garden variety poor reader: The phonological-core variable difference model. *Journal of Learning Disabilities* 21, 590–604.

Torgesen, J.K. (2005) Recent discoveries from research on remedial interventions for children with dyslexia. In M.J. Snowling and C. Hulme (eds) *The Science of Reading: A Handbook* (pp. 521–537). Malden, MA: Blackwell.

Tunmer, W.E. and Chapman, J. (1996) A developmental model of dyslexia. Can the construct be saved? *Dyslexia* 2, 179–189.

Usmani, K. (2000) The influence of racism and cultural bias in the assessment of bilingual children. *Educational and Child Psychology* 16, 44–54.

Ziegler, J., Bertrand, D., Tóth, D., Csépe, V., Reis, A., Faísca, L., Saine, N., Lyytinen, H., Vaessen, A. and Blomert, L. (2010) Orthographic depth and its impact on universal predictors of reading: A cross-language investigation. *Psychological Science* 21, 551–559.

2 Individual Differences in Learning a Foreign (Second) Language: A Cognitive Approach

Richard L. Sparks

Introduction

For over 20 years I and my colleague Leonore Ganschow have proposed that language aptitude and strengths and weaknesses in the components of language are important for understanding why some students learn a second language (L2) more easily than others. Both of us are special educators whose backgrounds are in learning disabilities and reading disabilities (dyslexia). Like cognitive psychology, the field of special education has a long history of studying individual differences among learners. In particular, researchers have found that the primary difference between good and poor readers is in phonological processing skills, that is, facility with speech sounds (phonemic awareness) and sound–symbol (phonological–orthographic) relationships (e.g. Rayner *et al.*, 2001; Snowling & Hulme, 2007). Our research with L2 learners in the USA has drawn heavily on research into reading, cognitive psychology, speech perception and learning disabilities (LD) in the native language (L1), and has shown consistently that there are differences in both L2 aptitude and the component skills of language – phonological, syntactic, semantic – between high- and low-achieving L2 learners. In addition, our studies indicate that individual differences in students' L2 aptitude and their L2 proficiency and achievement are related to individual differences in their L1 skills. Based on the results of our studies, we have proposed that individual differences in language skills play the primary role in students' L2 aptitude, proficiency and classroom achievement.

In this chapter I review research over 20 years that is informed by a cognitive approach to L2 learning. I review the paradigm we have used to conduct our investigations of L2 learning with US high school students. In this cognitive paradigm, I take the following positions: (1) L2 learning is the learning of *language*, that is, there is a talent (aptitude) specific to language learning; (2) language learning is special, that is, language learning is different from learning other skills, such as mathematics, rely on different cognitive skills to master their content; and (3) L2 aptitude is componential that is, composed of subskills in spoken and written language.

After reviewing the cognitive paradigm and evidence supporting these positions, I present a hypothesis that Ganschow and I have developed over many years of researching its basic premises, the Linguistic Coding Differences Hypothesis (LCDH). In this hypothesis, we propose that L1 skills are the foundation for L2 learning, and that individual differences in the subcomponents of language aptitude are likely to be the primary reason for high and low L2 proficiency and classroom achievement. We further speculate that while L2 students will exhibit individual differences in affective qualities, for example anxiety, in motivation and in personality variables, these differences are related generally to the efficiency of their language learning skills and are not the primary reason for good or poor L2 learning. Following my review of the LCDH and studies supporting its positions, I report on our recent longitudinal studies, both retrospective and prospective, which support the view that L2 aptitude and proficiency are strongly related to students' early levels of and individual differences in L1 skills, particularly L1 literacy. I conclude by raising the question of the cross-linguistic transfer of L1 to L2 learning and by citing implications for future research in L2 learning.

Cognitive Paradigm of L2 Learning

One reason for the lack of research relating to L2 aptitude is the disagreement about the assumption that language is special, that there is a talent (aptitude) specific to language learning (Skehan, 1998). Here, my position is different from researchers who view language learning ability as similar to the learning of other skills, for example mathematics, and who propose that the skills which facilitate language learning are the same as those in any other learning task. Their view implies that a high-achieving language learner will exhibit strong skills across academic subjects because of, for example, strong general intelligence and strong memory skills. In contrast, I take the position that students can have high general intelligence and strong memory skills but exhibit individual differences in specific subject areas (e.g. strong mathematics but weak reading and spelling), in subcomponents of language (e.g. strong grammar and oral vocabulary but weak phonological skills) and/or individual differences in the subcomponents of L2 aptitude (e.g. strong rote memory but weak grammar skills).

Support for the view that language is qualitatively different from other cognitive skills comes from studies with exceptional learners and the field of L1 reading, including students with LD and dyslexia. Studies with exceptional learners show a separation between language skills and other cognitive abilities. For example, Skehan (1998) reviews studies which have shown that there are: (1) exceptional L2 learners who have brain damage but demonstrate extraordinary talent for L2 learning; (2) exceptional learners who have low cognitive ability (IQ) but nevertheless demonstrate extraordinary language skills in one or more components of language; and (3) relatively unsuccessful L2 learners who have average to above-average cognitive ability but fail at L2 learning because of low aptitude in one or more components of language.

In L1 reading, evidence has shown that learning to read is a *language-related* skill (see reviews by Rayner *et al.*, 2001; Stanovich, 2000). Researchers have found consistently that students who are poor readers may exhibit strong skills in some areas, for example mathematics, because the skills that facilitate reading, for example phonological processing, grammar and morphology, are substantively different from those in other learning tasks, such as mathematics. Students with L1 reading difficulties have been called 'at risk' for L2 learning, and some have been classified as LD or dyslexic in their L1 (Nijakowska, 2010). I have extensively studied, with my colleagues, these 'at-risk' groups who exhibit L1 reading difficulties and found that, while they exhibit average cognitive ability (IQ) generally and average or better skills in other areas, for example mathematics, science and spatial ability, they consistently exhibit low L2 aptitude (on an L2 aptitude test), weak oral and written L2 proficiency, and poor L2 classroom achievement (see reviews by Ganschow & Sparks, 2001; Sparks, 2001).

Support for speculation that language is special also comes from studies with unique populations. In an investigation with exceptional learners who have very low cognitive ability but extraordinary L1 word reading ability, Sparks and Artzer (2000) studied three children with hyperlexia, each of whom read words spontaneously before the age of five and exhibited extraordinary word reading (decoding) skills but severely limited comprehension on both listening and reading tasks and well below average IQ. Hyperlexic children display very limited skills in all other areas of learning, including mathematics, science, vocabulary, spatial ability and general knowledge. Their strengths are word decoding and spelling that rely on strong phonological processing skills and these skills are well above their IQ (see Nation, 1999). After they had taken one year of foreign language (Spanish) in high school, the students received a comprehensive evaluation of their oral (listening, speaking) and written (word decoding, spelling, reading comprehension, writing) L2 proficiency. The results showed that all three students exhibited strong L2 word decoding skills that depended on intact phonological processing. But they showed severely limited L2 language comprehension (both reading and listening) and oral proficiency in Spanish, which depended on efficient use of grammar and semantics skills; that is, they were hyperlexic in both L1 and L2.

These findings support the views that language is special, that there is a talent specific to language learning, that there are skills that facilitate language learning which are different from those required for other learning tasks, and that language aptitude is componential.

Linguistic Coding Differences Hypothesis and Evidence for L1–L2 Connections

How does the cognitive paradigm assist us in understanding the relationship between L1 skills and L2 learning? Prior to our research with students who exhibit differences in L2 learning skills, some researchers had speculated that L1 skills are related to L2 aptitude and L2 learning. For example, John Carroll, author of the Modern Language Aptitude Test (MLAT) (Carroll & Sapon, 1959, 2001), speculated that L2 aptitude is a 'residue' of L1 learning skills (Carroll, 1973). Cummins (1979) developed the Linguistic Interdependence Hypothesis, in which he hypothesised that L1 and L2 are interdependent and require a common proficiency on the part of the learner, and also that success in L2 learning is dependent primarily on L1 skills developed prior to L2 exposure. In his Threshold Hypothesis, Cummins (1979) speculated that the level of L2 proficiency is moderated by one's level of attainment in L1. Skehan and Ducroquet (1988) conducted a study that supported both Carroll's 'residue' speculation and Cummins' hypotheses. They followed children who had participated in the Bristol Language Project (Wells, 1985), whose language skills had been tested at 15–60 months of age. They administered measures of L2 aptitude and L2 achievement when the children were 13–14 years old. The results showed that: (1) L1 development, particularly early vocabulary and comprehension skills, was significantly related to L2 achievement at age 13; (2) L1 comprehension and vocabulary were significantly related to L2 aptitude at age 13; and(3) L2 aptitude was significantly related to L2 oral and written achievement. Skehan and Ducroquet also reported that early literacy-based factors in L1, for example comprehension, grammar and vocabulary, influenced L2 skills several years later.

In the 1990s Leonore Ganschow and I developed the Linguistic Coding Differences Hypothesis (LCDH) to explain why students in L2 classes (modern foreign languages) exhibited differences in their L2 learning and achievement. The LCDH proposes that: (1) L2 learning is built upon L1 skills; (2) both L1 and L2 learning depend on language learning mechanisms that are similar in both languages; and (3) problems with one component of language, for example phonological processing, will have a negative effect on the learning of both L1 and L2 (Sparks, 1995; Sparks & Ganschow, 1993, 1995; Sparks et al., 1989). In support for the idea that language is special, we found that high- and low-achieving L2 learners did not exhibit differences in mathematics (e.g. Ganschow et al., 1991). But our studies showed that secondary and post-secondary L2 learners who exhibit significant differences in L1 skills, especially L1 literacy, also exhibit significant differences in L2 aptitude (on the MLAT), L2 oral and written proficiency, and L2 classroom achievement.

In the last two dozen years, we have conducted a variety of studies that have supported the LCDH. Our comparison studies among diverse groups of L2 learners indicate that high-achieving L2 learners exhibit stronger L1 word decoding, pseudo-word decoding, spelling and writing skills, and higher L2 aptitude than low-achieving L2 learners, even after controlling for IQ (e.g. Sparks et al., 1992a). Our studies with high- and low-achieving L2 learners show that the groups exhibit differences in their L1 phonological process-ing skills, namely word decoding and spelling, but not in L1 vocabulary, L1 comprehension and/or intelligence (e.g. Ganschow et al., 1991; Sparks et al., 1992b). In other studies, we found that high-achieving L2 learners with stronger L1 literacy skills and higher L2 aptitude exhibit stronger oral and written L2 proficiency (in Spanish, French or German) than low-achieving L2 learners (e.g. Sparks et al., 1998a, 1998b). In studies with students classi-fied as LD and low-achieving (non-LD) students in L2 classes, we found no differences between the groups in L1 skills, IQ, L2 aptitude, L2 proficiency and L2 classroom achievement; that is, the cognitive profiles of these two groups were identical but only one group had a diagnostic label (see reviews by Sparks, 2001, 2006a). Our prediction studies indicate that the best predictors of L2 proficiency and L2 classroom achievement are language-related, namely L1 literacy and L2 aptitude (e.g. Sparks et al., 1995, 1997b). Studies conducted by other researchers in alphabetic and non-alphabetic orthographies/languages have also supported the position that there are strong relationships between L1 and L2 skills in both school-age and college populations (e.g. Chung & Suk-Han Ho, 2010; Dufva & Voeten, 1999; Kahn-Horwitz et al., 2005, 2006; Meschyan & Hernandez, 2002; Service & Kohonen, 1995).

Affective characteristics

For many years, affective factors such as motivation (Gardner, 1990), anxiety (Horwitz et al., 1986), personality (Ehrman, 1990) and learning strategies (Oxford, 1990) have held a special place in the L2 field as explana-tions for good and poor L2 learning. Early on, we questioned the assumption that these variables play a primary role in L2 learning and took the position that, although affective variables are important for learning all tasks (not just L2), they are not likely to be causal factors in learning a second language. Instead, we speculated that students with low motivation or high levels of anxiety and lower L2 proficiency are likely to exhibit lower levels of L1 skills, especially in L1 literacy, and L2 aptitude (Sparks & Ganschow, 1991). For example, our investigations have shown that secondary and post-secondary L2 learners who self-report higher levels of anxiety on Horwitz's Foreign

Language Classroom Anxiety Scale (FLCAS) (Horwitz *et al.*, 1986) exhibit significantly lower L1 skills, L2 aptitude and L2 proficiency than students with lower levels of anxiety (Ganschow & Sparks, 1996; Ganschow *et al.*,1994; Sparks *et al.*, 1997a).

In a longitudinal study (discussed again later in the chapter), students who self-reported lower levels of motivation for L2 learning in high school exhibited lower levels of L1 skills as early as elementary school – many years before they encountered a L2 (Sparks *et al.*, 2009a). In another study, students who self-reported higher levels of anxiety for L2 learning in high school exhibited lower levels of L1 skills – literacy, vocabulary and listening comprehension – as early as the second grade, several years *before* they began L2 study (Sparks & Ganschow, 2007). In this investigation, the students' scores on all measures of L1 achievement in elementary school were negatively correlated with score on the FLCAS, which had been administered in high school. We proposed that if the self-report measures used by L2 researchers involving L2 motivation and anxiety were indeed tapping into a type of motivation for or anxiety specific to L2 learning, there would be no *a priori* reasons: (1) to expect differences in L1 skills several years before exposure to the L2; or (2) to find that affect for L2 learning is negatively correlated with L1 skills several years before students encountered an L2 in the school environment. Instead, we have taken the position that affective measures in L2 studies are likely to be reflecting, often correctly, students' perceptions of their language learning skills. That is, students who report lower levels of motivation for, or higher levels of anxiety about, L2 learning are those who have lower levels of L1 skills and L2 aptitude and who will ultimately achieve lower L2 proficiency than students with stronger L1 skills and higher L2 aptitude.

Teaching strategies

In addition to our research on affective characteristics and L2 learning, we have posited that teaching language learning strategies or teaching to students' learning styles cannot increase achievement in L2 learning, because these strategies are not specifically related to language learning. Language learning strategies are thought to be 'learning processes which are consciously selected by the learner' (Cohen, 1998: 4) and involve a number of skills, such as memory, cognitive, compensatory, affective, metacognitive and social skills. Oxford (1990) has proposed that language learning strategies can be taught to improve students' language proficiency. Likewise, L2 educators have suggested that teaching to learning styles – a style is defined as 'an individual's natural, habitual, and preferred way(s) of absorbing, processing, and retaining new information and skills' (Reid, 1995: viii) – is important for successful L2 learning. Both of these ideas are intuitively appealing to educators because they are thought to be unrelated to language aptitude (ability) and reflect their belief that teaching specific strategies or responding to individual styles will result in enhanced L2 proficiency and achievement. However, both learning strategies and learning styles theories have been found to have a host of conceptual problems and there are a myriad of difficulties when attempting to operationalise the definitions of *strategies* and *styles* (see Dörnyei, 2005; Pashler *et al.*, 2009; Skehan, 1991; Sparks, 2006b).

In sum, students' L1 skills are strongly related to their L2 aptitude, proficiency and achievement, and differences in the components of students' language aptitude lead to different L2 outcomes. In contrast, affective variables are unlikely to be the primary factor in more and less successful L2 learning. Researchers have not found that use of learning strategies and teaching to learning styles are effective in the teaching of L2. Instead, the close connections between L1 and L2 skills, particularly between L1 literacy and L2 aptitude and proficiency, raise the question of whether there is cross-linguistic transfer of L1 knowledge and skills to L2 learning, an idea that I examine in the next section.

Longitudinal Evidence for L1–L2 Connections from Retrospective Studies

Our initial studies measured students' L1 skills and L2 aptitude either shortly before or when they began L2 study in high school and then followed them over 1–2 years, at which time their L2 proficiency was measured and markers of L2 classroom achievement were obtained. Given that we were measuring L1 skills only when the participants were beginning L2 study, we saw the need for longitudinal investigations to determine whether students' L1 skills many years prior to engaging in L2 study were related to their L2 aptitude and L2 proficiency in high school.

In just such a retrospective study, 156 US high school students were followed over seven years from the fourth grade (age 9–10) until the end of the tenth grade (age 15–16), by which time they had completed two years of Spanish (Sparks *et al.*, 2008). The purpose of this study was to determine how accurately a battery of L1 and L2 testing instruments discriminated membership of four groups of L2 learners: (1) high-achieving students ($n = 49$) who had achieved grade A or B in each of two quarters of first-year Spanish; (2) low-achieving students ($n = 55$) who had achieved grade C, D or F in each of two quarters of first-year Spanish; (3) students classified as LD ($n = 30$), with reading and writing difficulties, who were receiving special education services and had an active Individual Education Program (IEP); and (4) students classified as attention deficit hyperactivity disorder (ADHD) ($n = 22$) according to DSM-IV criteria and who had an active section 504 plan.[1,2] The students' scores on measures of L1 literacy (reading, writing) in the fourth grade and eighth grade, and cognitive ability (IQ) in the sixth grade were collected from school records. Each student was administered a L2 aptitude test (MLAT), measures of L2 literacy (word decoding and spelling) and a self-report measure of L2 motivation adapted from the Attitude/Motivation Test Battery (AMTB; Gardner, 1985). We conducted a discriminant analysis (a statistical technique used to examine differences between two or more groups on several variables) to determine which of the aforementioned testing measures best discriminated the four groups of L2 learners. The results showed that measures of L1 literacy (fourth-grade reading, eighth-grade writing), L2 word decoding and three MLAT subtests (phonetic coding, grammar and rote memory) best discriminated the four groups. A follow-up analysis found that the majority of the LD students (60%) were best reclassified into the low-achieving group, and that 14% were reclassified as high-achieving learners. These findings showed that students classified as LD and both low- and high-achieving learners exhibited similar levels of L1 skills and L2 aptitude, suggesting that some students classified as LD did not exhibit deficits in either L1 skills or L2 aptitude. The results were consistent with the authors' findings about the strong connections between L1 skills, L2 aptitude and L2 proficiency, and also findings which have shown that low-achieving L2 learners and students classified as LD enrolled in L2 classes exhibit similar profiles of L1 skills, L2 aptitude and L2 achievement (see also Sparks, 2001, 2006a).

In a second study with these students, we added measures of L2 proficiency and L2 classroom tests and quizzes designed by the school's L2 department, and first- and second-year L2 grades to the analysis to determine the extent of differences among the four groups on the measures of L1 skills and L2 aptitude, and on these additional L2 measures (Sparks *et al.*, 2008). Because there were significant overall differences in IQ among the four groups favouring the high-achieving group, students' IQ scores were used as a covariate in all of the analyses. Even so, the findings revealed significant differences between the high- and low-achieving groups and the high-achieving and LD groups on all of the L1 measures and on L2 aptitude, L2 proficiency and L2 grades. There were few significant differences between the high-achieving and ADHD groups, a finding that was similar to previous studies with college students classified as ADHD (Sparks *et al.*, 2004, 2005). However, no differences were found between the low-achieving (non-LD) and the LD group on any of the L1 and L2 measures. As in our other studies, the results showed that there are individual differences among L2 learners in language skills, and also that students classified as LD exhibit cognitive profiles that are no different from those of low-achieving, non-disabled students.

In a third longitudinal study with a different population of L2 learners, we sought to determine whether specific clusters of L2 learners' cognitive and achievement profiles – three groups in this study, high-, average- and low-achieving learners – would emerge from a sample of high school students, each of whom had been followed for two years and had completed two years of L2 study (Sparks *et al.*, 2012). The students (*n* = 208) had participated in one of our previous studies and were chosen for this investigation because each had been administered similar measures of L1 skills, intelligence (IQ) and L2 aptitude (MLAT), as well as the same measure of L2 proficiency. We conducted a non-hierarchical cluster analysis in which the L2 proficiency measure was used as the external criterion variable. The results showed that students in each cluster achieved scores on the L1 measures that were similar to their scores on the L2 aptitude and L2 proficiency measures. That is, students in the high-achieving cluster achieved in the high-average to above-average range generally on all of the L1 and L2 measures (65th–95th percentile); students in the average-achieving cluster achieved in the average range on all measures (28th–73rd percentile); and students in the low-achieving cluster achieved in the average to below-average range on all measures (6th–45th percentile) (see Figure 2.1). The findings showed that students who achieve strong scores on measures of L1 skill also achieve strong scores on measures of L2 aptitude and L2 proficiency, and vice versa, with average students scoring between the high and low groups.

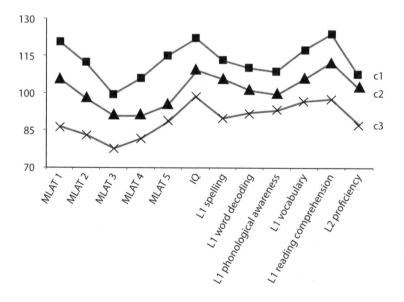

Figure 2.1 Plot of mean scores on L1 skill measures, L2 aptitude test (MLAT) and the L2 proficiency measures for the high-achieving (c1), average-achieving (c2) and low-achieving (c3) clusters

The results of these retrospective studies supported the findings of our earlier, short-term investigations, which had shown that students who exhibit strong L1 skills also have strong L2 aptitude and demonstrate strong L2 proficiency and classroom achievement. These findings are consistent with both Carroll's 'residue' speculation and Cummins' Linguistic Inter-dependence and Threshold Hypotheses as well as our LCDH, all of which propose that students' levels of L1 skills are related to the strength of their L2 aptitude and their subsequent levels of L2 oral and written proficiency. The findings raise important questions because they demonstrate the pos-sibility of long-term cross-linguistic transfer of L1 skills to L2 learning; they also highlight the importance of early L1 literacy skills for later L2 aptitude, proficiency and classroom achievement. The potential for investigating long-term, cross-linguistic transfer and the importance of early L1 skills for later L2 learning were the motivation for our next longitudinal study, which followed students over a 10-year period from first through to tenth grades.

Longitudinal Evidence for L1–L2 Connections from a 10-Year Prospective Study

In the early 1990s, Ganschow and I realised that the answers to questions we proposed about L2 learning – for example, are early L1 skills related to and predictive of later L2 aptitude and L2 proficiency? – could come only from an investigation that followed students from their earliest years of schooling until the time they completed L2 study in high school. Unlike Skehan and Ducroquet (1988), we did not have nor could we acquire a database of students who were followed before they began school. Therefore, we began a new prospective study in 1992 that followed three cohorts of students in one school district over 10 years, from first through to tenth grade.

The study began with 156 students in first grade who were enrolled in one elementary school in a large, rural school district. By the time the students in the three cohorts had reached ninth grade, when their L2 courses began, 77 students who had chosen to enrol in L2 courses remained in the district. Over the next two years of high school, 54 students completed the study by taking two years of high school L2 courses (Spanish $n = 30$, French $n = 14$, German $n = 10$). From the first through to the fifth grades, students were administered measures of L1 word decoding, spelling, vo-cabulary, phonemic awareness and reading comprehension. In the third and fifth grades, a measure of L1 listening comprehension was administered. Students' cognitive ability (IQ) scores were obtained from school records. At the beginning of the ninth grade, a measure of L2 aptitude (MLAT) was administered, along with a measure of L2 motivation (Gardner's AMTB). At the end of the ninth grade, an L2 anxiety survey (Horwitz et al.'s FLCAS) was administered to the participants. At the end of the tenth grade, participants were administered measures of oral (listening comprehension, oral expression) and written (word decoding, spelling, reading comprehension, writing) L2 proficiency. The L2 proficiency measures were designed according to guidelines from the American Council on the Teaching of Foreign Languages (ACTFL) and administered by L2 educators who were formally trained in ACTFL guidelines. Students' course grades in the first and second year of the L2 courses were obtained from school records.

In the first study we sought to determine the best L1 predictors of L2 aptitude (on the MLAT) and L2 oral and written proficiency (Sparks *et al.*, 2006). Here, we used the L1 skill measures administered in the first through to the fifth grades as predictor variables, to determine which measures would emerge as the best predictors of L2 aptitude and L2 proficiency. The statistical analysis showed that L1 reading, spelling, vocabulary and cognitive ability in elementary school accounted for 73% of the variance in L2 aptitude in the ninth grade; but the bulk of the variance was explained by L1 spelling and word decoding skills. Reading was a total score that included decoding and comprehension skills. L1 reading skill in elementary school alone explained 40% of the variance in L2 proficiency at the end of the tenth grade. These findings provided support for long-term connections between early L1 skills and later L2 aptitude and proficiency.

In a second study we conducted a series of multiple regression analyses to determine whether early L1 reading and spelling skills would predict later L2 reading and spelling skills (Sparks *et al.*, 2008). In this study, the measures of L1 word decoding, spelling, reading comprehension, phonological awareness, vocabulary and listening comprehension administered in the first through to the fifth grades were used as predictors of L2 word decoding, reading comprehension and spelling at the end of the tenth grade. The best predictor of L2 word decoding skill in high school was L1 word decoding in elementary school, and the best predictor of later L2 spelling was L1 spelling in elementary school. The best predictor of L2 reading comprehension was L1 reading comprehension in elementary school. However, when L2 word decoding skill replaced L1 word decoding as a predictor variable for L2 reading comprehension in the analysis, the findings showed that L2 word decoding explained over 40% of the variance in comprehension. These findings suggested that even several years after students learn to read and spell in L1, word decoding, spelling and reading comprehension skills may transfer from L1 to L2.

In a third study, we examined the notion of long-term cross-linguistic transfer from L1 to L2 by dividing the 54 students into high-, average- and low-proficiency L2 groups, based on their performance on the L2 proficiency measure that had been administered in the tenth grade, and then comparing the three groups on the L1 achievement measures administered in elementary school, the L2 aptitude test (MLAT) and L2 course grades (Sparks *et al.*, 2009a). There were significant overall differences among the three proficiency groups on all of the L1 achievement measures (from second through to fifth grades), the MLAT, L2 word decoding and spelling, and L2 grades after the first and second years of the course. High-proficiency L1 learners exhibited stronger L1 skills, L2 aptitude and L2 word decoding and spelling skills, and also higher L2 course grades than the average- and low-proficiency learners. L1 skill differences emerged early in elementary school and were related to L2 aptitude, L2 proficiency and L2 achievement several years later in high school and provided strong support for long-term cross-linguistic transfer of L1 skills to L2.

In a fourth study, we examined the relationships among L1 skills, L2 aptitude, L2 proficiency and affective variables (Sparks *et al.*, 2009b). In this investigation, we were interested in the roles played by these variables in predicting L2 proficiency. The predictor variables for L2 proficiency included not only the L1 skills measured in elementary school but also IQ, L2 aptitude (MLAT) and L2 affective variables (motivation, anxiety) because we sought to determine which types of variables, language or affective, would best predict students' oral and written L2 proficiency. There were strong correlations between early L1 skills and later L2 proficiency, for example 0.64 for L1 word decoding, 0.68 for L1 spelling and 0.66 for L1 reading comprehension. However, the MLAT was the best predictor of overall L2 proficiency and most of the L2 proficiency subtests, with the exception of L2 word decoding. There was a strong correlation between the students' scores on the MLAT and their overall L2 proficiency (0.75). Early L1 skills, L2 motivation or L2 anxiety added a small amount of variance to the prediction of L2 proficiency. However, findings from this study and those described earlier suggested that the L1 motivation and L2 anxiety surveys were likely to be measuring students' self-perceptions of their language learning skills, not a specific motivation for or anxiety about L2 learning. Overall, the findings showed that language-related variables, in this case L2 aptitude, are the most robust predictors of L1 proficiency and suggested the possibility of long-term cross-linguistic transfer of early L1 skills to later L2 aptitude and L2 proficiency.

In the fifth investigation, we conducted a factor analysis that included all of the testing measures used in the study: L1 skills, IQ, L2 aptitude (the five MLAT subtests), L2 motivation and L2 anxiety (Sparks *et al.*, 2011). In this study, we wanted to determine whether L1 and L2 tests that measured similar language components, for example phonetic coding and grammar, would load on similar factors. The analysis yielded four factors: (1) language analysis, composed of L1 and L2 language comprehension, grammar and vocabulary measures, and inductive language learning subtests from the MLAT; (2) phonology/orthography, composed of L1 and L2 phonemic coding and phonological processing measures; (3) IQ/memory, composed of intelligence and the paired-associate learning subtest from the MLAT; and (4) self-perceptions of language skills, composed of the L2 motivation and L2 anxiety surveys. The four factors explained 76% of the variance in oral and written L2 proficiency, with the first three factors listed here accounting for the bulk of the variance. The results showed that L1 phonological processing skills (word decoding, spelling, phonological awareness) loaded on the same factor as L2 phonological skills (MLAT phonetic script, MLAT spelling clues) and also that L1 language comprehension, vocabulary and reading comprehension skills loaded on the same factor as L2 grammar and language comprehension skills (MLAT word in sentences, MLAT number learning). The findings supported the claim that language aptitude is componential and can be divided into subcomponents, each of which makes a contribution to language learning.

Each of the investigations from this 10-year longitudinal study supports the primary tenets of the LCDH: (1) L2 learning is built on L1 learning; (2) L1 and L2 depend on language mechanisms that are similar in both languages; and (3) problems with one component (subskill) of language has a negative effect on both L1 and L2 learning. Our studies lend further credibility to Carroll's 'residue' speculation, which would suggest that L2 aptitude is, in part, a residue of L1 learning skills, and Cummins' Linguistic Interdependence Hypothesis, which would suggest that L1 and L2 have a common underlying proficiency, as well as Cummins' Threshold Hypothesis, which would suggest that the level of L2 proficiency is moderated by the level of attainment in L1. Our results also support Skehan and Ducroquet, whose study found strong relationships between early L1 skills and later L2 aptitude and achievement.

Taken together, the aforementioned studies are consistent with the claims of the cognitive paradigm for L2 learning: (1) L2 learning is the learning of language; (2) language learning is special and is different from other skills such as mathematics; and (3) language aptitude is componential and comprises specific subskills that make separate contributions to language learning.

Summary and Implications for a Future Research Agenda

In a recent ACTFL paper, 'We ignore research at our own peril', Rex (2011) posits that most L2 textbook publishers have ignored the results of recent research when designing language teaching curricula. As a special educator who has researched L2 learning for over 20 years, I take the position that many L2 educators and researchers have not taken advantage of the recent research on individual differences in language learning in the L1 and L2 fields. To a large extent, L2 educators and researchers have assumed that L2 learners have similar language learning potential and will learn through similar teaching approaches. As a result, they have not considered the importance of examining individual differences in language learning. In my view, these assumptions are misguided because they fail to take into account recent research described in this chapter, which has shown that L2 learners exhibit differences in language aptitude (potential) and language skills (components). How might L2 educators and researchers use cognitive research and re-examine long-held positions about L2 learning?

First, L2 educators should devise pedagogic approaches which support the claims that language is special and that students exhibit individual differences in language learning. For example, some students come into the L2 classroom with strong skills in the phonology and grammar of their L1, while some students still have not mastered all of the letter–sound relationships and grammatical structures in the language they have been speaking, reading and writing for years. When conducting research in L2 classrooms, I hear constantly what I call the L2 teacher's lament: How can I teach them grammar and spelling in, for example, Spanish, when they don't know English grammar and can't spell English words very well? In the L1 literature, there is abundant empirical evidence that students display individual differences in the components of language and that these differences either foster or hinder L1 language learning. Likewise, recent evidence in the L2 literature has shown that both language aptitude and individual differences in language components are strongly related to L2 proficiency and achievement. L2 pedagogy could take advantage of this research and use it to develop methods that attend to students' individual differences in language skills. Likewise, L2 researchers who contend that language aptitude and language strengths/weaknesses are unimportant for L2 proficiency should reconsider their assumptions and conduct studies on the relationships among L1 skills, L2 aptitude and L2 proficiency.

Second, L2 pedagogy could further examine the role that affective characteristics, such as anxiety and motivation, play in L2 learning. The notion that affective differences are causal variables is problematic for several reasons, most notably because affective characteristics such as low motivation and high levels of anxiety are *not* directly related to language learning. Affective characteristics are not unimportant for L2 learning, but there is no reason to think that motivation and anxiety are somehow more important for L2 learning than for other academic tasks. The question for L2 pedagogy concerns whether low motivation for or high anxiety about L2 learning is the result of problems with low skills in one or more language components, for example phonology or grammar. The research presented here shows that low motivation and high levels of anxiety for L2 learning are linked to significantly lower levels of L1 skills as early as primary school, several years *before* exposure to L2 instruction. Given such findings, there are reasons for L2 pedagogy to focus less on students' perceived motivation and anxiety in the L2 classroom and more on what the students know and need to learn about language to enhance L2 learning.

Third, research in L2 pedagogy could examine assumptions that teaching learning strategies and teaching to learning styles are important in increasing L2 proficiency. The idea of teaching learning strategies has been popular for many years but has not been supported in either the L1 or the L2 literature. Moreover, teaching to a student's learning style, for example auditory versus visual, analytical versus holistic, has been thoroughly debunked by L1 research (see Pashler *et al.*, 2009; Sparks, 2006b) and has not generated support in the L2 research literature (see Dörnyei, 2005). On the other hand, there is some empirical support for the recommendation that teaching language skills directly and explicitly, especially to students with language learning problems and to low-achieving L2 learners, is helpful in increasing L2 proficiency and achievement (Demuth & Smith, 1987; Downey & Snyder, 2001; Sparks *et al.*, 1999b).

Fourth, recent teaching recommendations have emphasised that the most important task for the L2 learner is to understand and communicate meaning. In the communicative approach, students are generally not taught directly and explicitly the components of language, for example grammar; instead, they are encouraged to negotiate meaning through interaction in the target language. Notwithstanding its widespread use in language teaching curricula, there has been little empirical research that compares the L2 competence (proficiency) of students who are taught by the communicative approach with the competence of students who are taught through other approaches to language teaching. Communicative approaches to L2 learning are similar to the whole-language method for teaching L1 reading, which has been popular among educators. Whole-language proponents take the position that learning to read an L1 is as natural as learning to perceive and produce speech (e.g. Goodman, 1973). Thus, the components of language – phonology, grammar, vocabulary, morphology – are not taught directly and explicitly (Liberman & Liberman, 1990). However, voluminous evidence accumulated over 30 years has shown that efficient word recognition, which is dependent on phonological processing skills, is best taught by direct teaching of sound–symbol relationships (e.g. National Reading Panel, 2000). Likewise, the ability to spell and knowledge of grammar are necessary for effective written communication and are learned through direct instruction. In the USA, the explicit teaching of letter–sound relationships (i.e. phonics) has been reintroduced into reading curricula. Like research has been done on the learning of L1 reading, I would argue that L2 researchers should conduct empirical studies to determine whether the communicative approach is more effective in promoting L2 oral and written proficiency than other teaching methods that teach L2 skills directly and explicitly.

A future agenda for researching L2 learning difficulties could examine L2 learning in the context of the premises promoted by the cognitive paradigm that have been supported by empirical research presented in this chapter.

Notes

1   Students who are provided with an Individualized Educational Program (IEP) by the school district are those who have been diagnosed with a disability under the Individuals with Disabilities Education Act (IDEA). An IEP provides the student with an 'appropriate education program', that is, with special education services (e.g. special education class) and other related services (e.g. testing accommodations) (deBettencourt, 2002).
2   Students who are provided with a 504 plan by the school district are those who qualify for related services (e.g. testing accommodations) but not special education services, under section 504 of the Rehabilitation Act (deBettencourt, 2002).

References

Carroll, J. (1973) Implications of aptitude test research and psycholinguistic theory for foreign language learning. *International Journal of Psycholinguistics* 2, 5–14.

Carroll, J. and Sapon, S. (1959, 2000) *Modern Language Aptitude Test (MLAT): Manual.* San Antonio, TX: Psychological Corp. Republished by Second Language Testing. See http://www.2LTI.com (accessed June 2013).

Chung, K. and Suk-Han Ho, C. (2010) Second language learning difficulties in Chinese children with dyslexia: What are the reading-related cognitive skills that contribute to English and Chinese word reading? *Journal of Learning Disabilities* 43, 195–211.

Cohen, A. (1998) *Strategies in Learning and Using a Second Language.* Harlow: Longman.

Cummins, J. (1979) Linguistic interdependence and educational development of bilingual children. *Review of Educational Research* 49, 222–251.

deBettencourt, L. (2002) Understanding the difference between IDEA and section 504. *Teaching Exceptional Children* 34, 16–23.

Demuth, K. and Smith, N. (1987) The foreign language requirement: An alternative program. *Foreign Language Annals* 20, 67–77.

Dörnyei, Z. (2005) *The Psychology of the Language Learner: Individual Differences in Second Language Acquisition.* Hillsdale, NJ: Erlbaum.

Downey, D. and Snyder, L. (2001) Curricular accommodations for college students with language learning disabilities. *Topics in Language Disorders* 21, 55–67.

Dufva, M. and Voeten M. (1999) Native language literacy and phonological memory as prerequisites for learning English as a foreign language. *Applied Psycholinguistics* 20, 329–348.

Ehrman, M. (1990) The role of personality type in adult language learning: An ongoing investigation. In T. Parry and C. Stansfield (eds) *Language Aptitude Reconsidered* (pp. 126–176). Englewood Cliffs, NJ: Prentice-Hall.

Ganschow, L. and Sparks, R. (1996) Foreign language anxiety among high school women. *Modern Language Journal* 80, 199–212.

Ganschow, L. and Sparks, R. (2001) Learning difficulties and foreign language learning: A review of research and instruction. *Language Teaching* 34, 79–98.

Ganschow, L., Sparks, R., Javorsky, J., Pohlman, J. and Bishop-Marbury, A. (1991) Identifying native language difficulties among foreign language learners in college: A foreign language learning disability? *Journal of Learning Disabilities* 24, 530–541.

Ganschow, L., Sparks, R., Anderson, R., Javorsky, J., Skinner, S. and Patton, J. (1994) Differences in anxiety and language performance among high, average, and low anxious college foreign language learners. *Modern Language Journal* 78, 41–55.

Gardner, R. (1985) *The Attitude/Motivation Test Battery: Technical Report.* London, Ontario: University of Western Ontario.

Gardner, R. (1990) Attitudes, motivation, and personality as predictors of success in foreign language learning. In T. Parry and C. Stansfield (eds) *Language Aptitude Reconsidered* (pp. 179–221). Englewood Cliffs, NJ: Prentice-Hall.

Goodman, K. (1973) Psycholinguistic universals of the reading process. In F. Smith (ed.) *Psycholinguistics and Reading* (pp. 1–29). New York: Holt, Rinehart, and Winston.

Horwitz, E., Horwitz, M. and Cope, J. (1986) Foreign language classroom anxiety. *Modern Language Journal* 70, 125–132.

Kahn-Horwitz, J., Shimron, J. and Sparks, R. (2005) Predicting foreign language reading achievement in elementary school students. *Reading and Writing: An Interdisciplinary Journal* 18, 527–558.

Kahn-Horwitz, J., Shimron, J. and Sparks, R. (2006) Weak and strong novice readers of English as a foreign language: Effects of first language and socioeconomic status. *Annals of Dyslexia* 56, 161–185.

Liberman, I. and Liberman, A. (1990) Whole language vs. code emphasis: Underlying assumptions and their implications for reading instruction. *Annals of Dyslexia* 40, 51–76.

Meschyan, G. and Hernandez, A. (2002) Is native-language decoding skill related to second-language learning? *Journal of Educational Psychology* 94, 14–22.

Nation, K. (1999) Reading skills in hyperlexia: A developmental perspective. *Psychological Bulletin* 125, 338–355.

National Reading Panel (2000) *Teaching Children to Read: An Evidence-Based Assessment of the Scientific Research Literature on Reading and Its Implications for Reading Instruction.* Washington, DC: National Instuitute for Child Health and Human Development.

Nijakowska, J. (2010) *Dyslexia in the Foreign Language Classroom.* Bristol: Multilingual Matters.

Oxford, R. (1990) Styles, strategies, and aptitude: Connections for language learning. In T. Parry and C. Stansfield (eds) *Language Aptitude Reconsidered* (pp. 67–125). Englewood Cliffs, NJ: Prentice-Hall.

Pashler, H., McDaniel, M., Rohrer, D. and Bjork, R. (2009) Learning styles: Concepts and evidence. *Psychological Science in the Public Interest* 9 (3), 105–119.

Rayner, K., Foorman, B., Perfetti, C., Pesetsky, D. and Seidenberg, M. (2001) How psychological science informs the teaching of reading. *Psychological Science in the Public Interest* 2, 31–74.

Reid, J. (1995) Preface. In J. Reid (ed.) *Learning Styles in the ESL/EFL Classroom* (pp. viii–xvii. Boston, MA: Heinle and Heinle.

Rex, S. (2011) We ignore current language research at our peril. *Language Educator* 6, 40–41.

Service, E. and Kohonen, V. (1995) Is the relation between phonological memory and foreign language learning accounted for by vocabulary acquisition? *Applied Psycholinguistics* 16, 155–172.

Skehan, P. (1991) Individual differences in second language learning. *Studies in Second Language Acquisition* 13, 275–298.

Skehan, P. (1998) *A Cognitive Approach to Language Learning.* Oxford: Oxford University Press.

Skehan, P. and Ducroquet, L. (1988) *A Comparison of First and Foreign Language Ability* (Working Documents No. 8). ESOL Department, Institute of Education, London University.

Snowling, M. and Hulme, C. (2007) *The Science of Reading: A Handbook.* Malden, MA: Blackwell.

Sparks, R. (1995) Examining the linguistic coding differences hypothesis to explain individual differences in foreign language learning. *Annals of Dyslexia* 45, 187–214.

Sparks, R. (2001) Foreign language learning problems of students classified as learning disabled and non-learning disabled: Is there a difference? *Topics in Language Disorders* 21, 38–54.

Sparks, R. (2006a) Is there a 'disability' for learning a foreign language? *Journal of Learning Disabilities* 39, 544–557.

Sparks, R. (2006b) Learning styles – making too many 'wrong mistakes': A response to Castro and Peck. *Foreign Language Annals* 39, 520–528.

Sparks, R. and Artzer, M. (2000) Foreign language learning, hyperlexia, and early word recognition. *Annals of Dyslexia* 50, 189–211.

Sparks, R. and Ganschow, L. (1991) Foreign language learning difficulties: Affective or native language aptitude differences? *Modern Language Journal* 75, 3–16.

Sparks, R. and Ganschow, L. (1993) Searching for the cognitive locus of foreign language learning problems: Linking first and second language learning. *Modern Language Journal* 77, 289–302.

Sparks, R. and Ganschow, L. (1995) A strong inference approach to causal factors in foreign language learning: A response to MacIntyre. *Modern Language Journal* 79, 235–244.

Sparks, R. and Ganschow, L. (2007) Is the Foreign Language Classroom Anxiety Scale measuring anxiety or language skills? *Foreign Language Annals* 40, 260–287.

Sparks, R., Ganschow, L. and Pohlman, J. (1989) Linguistic coding deficits in foreign language learners. *Annals of Dyslexia* 39, 179–195.

Sparks, R., Ganschow, L., Javorsky, J., Pohlman, J. and Patton, J. (1992a) Identifying native language deficits in high- and low-risk foreign language learners in high school. *Foreign Language Annals* 25, 403–418.

Sparks, R., Ganschow, L., Javorsky, J., Pohlman, J. and Patton, J. (1992b) Test comparisons among hi-risk, low-risk, and learning disabled students enrolled in foreign language courses. *Modern Language Journal* 76, 142–159.

Sparks, R., Ganschow, L. and Patton, J. (1995) Prediction of performance in first-year foreign language courses: Connections between native and foreign language learning. *Journal of Educational Psychology* 87, 638–655.

Sparks, R., Ganschow, L., Artzer, M., Siebenhar, D. and Plageman, M. (1997a) Anxiety and proficiency in a foreign language. *Perceptual and Motor Skills* 85, 559–562.

Sparks, R., Ganschow, L., Patton, J., Artzer, M., Siebenhar, D. and Plageman, M. (1997b) Prediction of foreign language proficiency. *Journal of Educational Psychology* 89, 549–561.

Sparks, R., Artzer, M., Javorsky, J., Patton, J., Ganschow, L., Miller, K. and Hordubay, D. (1998a) Students classified as learning disabled (LD) and non learning disabled students: Two comparison studies of native language skill, foreign language aptitude, and foreign language proficiency. *Foreign Language Annals* 31, 531–551.

Sparks, R., Artzer, M., Patton, J., Ganschow, L., Miller, K., Hordubay, D. and Walsh, G. (1998b) Benefits of multisensory language instruction in Spanish for at-risk learners: A comparison study of high school Spanish students. *Annals of Dyslexia* 48, 239–270.

Sparks, R., Ganschow, L., Artzer, M., Siebenhar, D. and Plageman, M. (1998c) Differences in native language skills, foreign language aptitude, and foreign language grades among high, average, and low proficiency learners: Two studies. *Language Testing* 15, 181–216.

Sparks, R., Javorsky, J. and Philips, L. (2004) College students classified with attention deficit hyperactivity disorder (ADHD) and the foreign language requirement. *Journal of Learning Disabilities* 37, 169–178.

Sparks, R., Javorsky, J. and Philips, L. (2005) Comparison of the performance of college students classified as ADHD, LD, and LD/ADHD in foreign language courses. *Language Learning* 55, 151–177.

Sparks, R., Patton, J., Ganschow, L., Humbach, N. and Javorsky, J. (2006) Native language predictors of foreign language proficiency and foreign language aptitude. *Annals of Dyslexia* 56, 129–160.

Sparks, R., Ganschow, L. and Patton, J. (2008a) L1 and L2 literacy, aptitude, and affective variables as discriminators among high and low-achieving L2 learners. In J. Kormos and E. Kontra (eds) *Language Learners with Special Needs: An International Perspective* (pp. 11–35). London: Multilingual Matters.

Sparks, R., Humbach, N. and Javorsky, J. (2008b) Comparing high and low achieving, LD, and ADHD foreign language learners: Individual and longitudinal differences. *Learning and Individual Differences* 18, 29–43.

Sparks, R., Patton, J., Ganschow, L., Humbach, N. and Javorsky, J. (2008c) Early first-language reading and spelling skills predict later second-language reading and spelling skills. *Journal of Educational Psychology* 100, 162–174.

Sparks, R., Patton, J., Ganschow, L. and Humbach, N. (2009a) Long-term cross linguistic transfer of skills from L1 to L2. *Language Learning* 59, 203–243.

Sparks, R., Patton, J., Ganschow, L. and Humbach, N. (2009b) Long-term relationships among early language skills, L2 aptitude, L2 affect, and later L2 proficiency. *Applied Psycholinguistics* 30, 725–755.

Sparks, R., Patton, J., Ganschow, L. and Humbach, N. (2011) Subcomponents of second-language aptitude and second-language proficiency. *Modern Language Journal* 95, 1–21.

Sparks, R., Patton, J. and Ganschow, L. (2012) Profiles of more and less successful L2 learners: A cluster analysis study. *Learning and Individual Differences* 22, 463–472.

Stanovich, L. (2000) *Progress in Understanding Reading: Scientific Foundations and New Frontiers*. New York: Guilford.

Wells, G. (1985) *Language Development in the Pre-school Years*. London: Cambridge University Press.

3 Cognitive Intervention to Enhance Foreign Language Reading Comprehension in Adolescents With Dyslexia Difficulties

Carol Goldfus

Introduction

Understanding language-related disabilities in the multilingual society of modern times has undergone many changes (McGill-Franzen & Allington, 2011). Until recently, the field of dyslexia was placed within the framework of special education and intervention meant helping children to learn how to read. Reading disabilities, however, are found not just within those educational settings of special education but also in the typical classroom and relate not only to learning to read but reading to learn in more than one language.

Not every teacher need be an expert in assessment, but every teacher ought to have enough knowledge to profile those pupils with difficulties, understand the different kinds of difficulties that may occur and build intervention programmes that will enable most pupils to overcome their difficulties and to succeed.

Learning a language in educational contexts is likely to require the learning of literacy skills. Literacy in schooling is understood mainly as an independent, autonomous set of skills for reading and writing words and texts. Literacy skills include the ability to process information, to understand written text and to write clearly and coherently; it 'involves more than decoding' (Westby, 2002: 73). In the light of technological development, communication and the information explosion of the 21st century, the field of new literacy studies has expanded the notion of literacies to be more than technical skills in reading and writing. Literacies and literacy practices include the ability to create something to communicate and to understand what others have created (Mayer, 2008).

This chapter addresses from a cognitive processing perspective intervention in reading comprehension for those adolescent pupils who do not succeed in the academic setting. I present an intervention approach to address substantial difficulties in developing literacy skills with adolescents aged 16–18, in secondary school, who have experienced failure in learning literacy skills in a second/foreign language for some time. The approach adopts a cognitive understanding of learning literacy skills and a cognitive interpretation of difficulties in reading and literacy skills. The theoretical basis of the intervention programme, its key principles and the main features of its implementation are discussed and illustrated across three levels of reading skills: word, intrasentential and intersentential.

Researching Language-Related Disabilities

This section begins with issues in terminology and measurement that make it difficult for researchers to reach an agreement about the meaning of the term 'dyslexia'. It goes on to discuss the cognitive process involved in reading.

The term 'learning disabilities' refers to a heterogeneous group of language-related difficulties which express themselves in the acquisition and effective use of speech, listening, reading, writing and mathematics (Gunderson & D'Silva, 2011: 14, 15). There are various degrees of severity of these difficulties. The term 'dyslexia' specifically refers to difficulties experienced by pupils in learning to read and reaching automaticity in acquiring learning (Goldfus, 2010) and students who are slower to learn in comparison with peers and find that they need to put more effort into their work than their peers (Nicolson & Fawcett, 2008; Shaywitz, 2003). Dyslexia is called the 'hidden disability' (Shaywitz, 2003: 4) as there are no external features which point to the problem, with the result that many educationists and others do not notice the specificity of difficulty with literacy skills.

Most research to date has focused on elementary school children in the early stages of learning literacy skills, on decoding skills and on word reading and retrieval, and is conducted on English as a mother tongue. Recently, however, a research focus has been on difficulties in learning literacy skills in orthographies and languages other than English. In addition, most research on decoding, phonological processing and word recognition adopts quantitative methodologies and methods. This is reflected, too, in most of the research on the learning of a foreign language (Sparks et al., 2002; and Chapter 2 of this book).

It may be easier to notice and identify difficulties when students read aloud but it is more difficult to understand what is going on in the mind of the reader during silent reading of a text. One of the limitations in the field of research into learning difficulties is the scarcity of norms for measuring comprehension. The participants in most of the research have been around the age of 12. The intervention programme discussed here concerns adolescent pupils with difficulties, aged 16–18, in secondary school, and focuses on the complex cognitive processes needed for reading comprehension. Other aspects of literacy skills, such as spelling and writing, are not dealt with here.

Looking specifically at the reading process from a cognitive psychological perspective, reading is a multifaceted, complex set of skills that involves a number of component operations, each dependent on and the product of a wide range of competencies (Cutting *et al.*, 2009; Ghelani *et al.*, 2004; Koda, 2005). It is the complex process of problem solving in which the reader works to make sense of a text not just from the words and sentences on the page, but also from the ideas, memories and knowledge evoked by those words and sentences. Reading involves many complex skills that have come together in order for the reader to read successfully.

From one perspective, reading in a second language is seen as additionally difficult. The complexity of reading increases in English as another language since, by definition, reading involves more than one language. Critical within the second/foreign language framework is the fact that 'readers approach a text from their first language framework. Hence, a conflict exists from the micro-level features of text through grammatical structures' (Bernhardt, 1993: 16). This situation is exacerbated in the foreign language situation. If difficulties have arisen in the acquisition of the mother tongue (L1), this will also be found in reading comprehension in another language (L2). The term 'second/foreign language' assumes that one language has already been acquired. In this case difficulties in the one language manifest themselves in another language. This has been shown in recent research (Sparks *et al.*, 2009; and see Chapter 2) where it was shown that literacy skills in L1 could account for individual differences in L2 learning and that proficiency in L1 was a strong indicator of successful learning of the second language.

Reading Difficulties

In this section I review literature on literacy difficulties, specifically studies of word-level, intrasentential and intersentential reading difficulties.

Difficulties reading at the word level are a fundamental concern. Word level 'is a baseline against which to assess the role of higher-level processes, such as comprehension monitoring and inference making' (Perfetti *et al.*, 2005: 242; see also Perfetti *et al.*, 1996).

Studies reveal that another level of difficulty in reading is failure to understand certain grammatical constructions (Oakhill & Yuill, 1996; Vellutino & Fletcher, 2005). That is, poor comprehension by first language and foreign language students may be due to their tendency to read word by word, rather than processing the text in larger grammatical units that are more meaningful. This difficulty constructing meaning intrasententially has implications for processing the next sentence for intersentential meaning. This is where breakdown occurs. Students who do not or cannot use the sentence and text structure to guide them will not understand what they read.

Reading comprehension difficulties can occur at text level. Developing a mental model of the main points of the paragraph/passage and inference play an important role in reading comprehension of texts (Schmalhofer & Perfetti, 2007). The extent to which information is integrated into a coherent 'text model' (Grabe, 2009: 206) and the extent to which inference is used to do this distinguish skilled readers from both less skilled readers and at-risk learners (Perfetti, 1994; Perfetti et al., 2005; Yuill & Oakhill, 1991). Less-skilled comprehenders have difficulty taking advantage of the cohesive links in a text (Kintsch & Rawson, 2005). Explanations include either that they do not realise that inferential processing is necessary or relevant to understanding the passages, or that they have difficulty in accessing the relevant knowledge and integrating it with the information in the text. These difficulties may arise because these learners have cognitive processing limitations. Research has found that students with difficulties understanding/reading texts cannot be accounted for in terms of word-decoding difficulties (Perfetti, 1994; Vellutino & Fletcher, 2005). Their difficulties relate to being able to judge what is important in a body of text. Their difficulties in understanding what they have read indicate a less integrated idea of what the passage is about. The students have distinct difficulties in processing a text.

Moving away from word, sentence and text levels of print, another source of difficulty for these learners is metacognition.

Metacognition refers to one's knowledge concerning one's own cognitive processes or anything related to them, e.g. the learning-relevant properties of information or data. For example, I am engaging in metacognition if I notice that I am having more trouble learning A than B; if it strikes me that I should double check C before accepting it as fact. (Flavell, 1976: 232)

Difficulties in this area manifest themselves in many ways. 'Poor comprehenders' is a term used to describe this group (Oakhill & Garnham, 1988). They tend to be less aware of their own lack of understanding. They have difficulty in being able to assess the ease or difficulty of the passage, and cannot explain why a text is difficult (Butler, 1998; Ehrlich, 1996; Garner, 1987; Oakhill & Yuill, 1996). In monitoring their understanding of a text, poor comprehenders are more concerned with individual words than the text as a whole. Comprehension monitoring, that is, awareness of understanding, is not developed. Indeed, they expect not to understand. Further, these students emphasise accurate decoding rather than attending to the meaning of the text. In the foreign language situation, when asked what they are currently learning, based on my observations in teaching, the answer is usually a grammatical structure (e.g. present simple).

Further explanations in a cognitive approach for reading comprehension difficulties may lie in memory resources. Long-term memory is needed for storage, relevant background and for making inferences (Randall, 2007). The demands on working memory in the processing of language may lead to overload, that is, demands to process information outstrip the reader's memory resources, so that storage of the information is not carried over to long-term memory resources. The point of difficulty here is that simultaneous storage and processing demands on working memory may be dysfunctional. Consequently reading comprehension problems may arise as a result of incorrect processing of information in memory. The findings reported in this area relate to experimental studies that aimed to explore the problematic of reading comprehension. An important consideration for intervention research is the extent to which these difficulties are considered permanent and impermeable, or whether they can be shown to be responsive to appropriate teaching. The intervention programme presented here addresses these difficulties in both languages of the learners and teachers, namely, the mother tongue and the foreign language, in this case English as the foreign (second) language.

To fully understand the intended meaning of a passage that has been read, the reader needs to go beyond that which is explicitly stated, to draw on other knowledge that is implied in the text and inferred by the reader. Furthermore, I argue that the strengths of the adolescent students with dyslexia should be reinforced in order to help them cope with their weaknesses. Meaning and semantics, which in the mother tongue is usually intact in learning-disabled students (Ganschow *et al.*, 1998), are the starting point for this intervention programme in L2, so that difficulties can be addressed. Cognitive intervention can take place and the process can be completed by returning to the aspect of meaning. This process is viewed as iterative.

Intervention

Intervention is referred to by different terms. In Britain, the term 'remediation' was used until the 1960s. In the current literature, the term used in British publications is 'intervention', whereas in US publications both 'remediation' and 'intervention' are used. Here, the preferred term is 'intervention' – a specific intervention for a specific problem. Intervention facilitates a change in cognitive and language functioning so as to produce changes in the way the learner relates to and copes with written material. Learners with learning disability may engage in many kinds of intervention at new learning stages in order to reach their desired objective, that is, being able to do the same work as their peers, and to meet their own needs. Intervention programmes need to consider how to enable at-risk students to start at their own level, evaluate their abilities and knowledge and understand the different aspects of reading. In addition, they need to help learners to be able to check themselves against their learning target and to assess their progress.

The intervention programme presented in this chapter is intended for the adolescent learner, aged 15–18 years (in the 9th to 12th grades), where the requirements demand that they reach a high level of reading proficiency. It assumes previous teaching about decoding as well as many attempts at learning to read English as a foreign language. The method described here emphasises *reading for understanding* in order to meet external requirements rather than reading at the decoding stage (learning to read). Special attention is paid to the ability of the learner to transfer from the specific teaching/ learning task to the more general learning goal. It assumes learners have a low frustration threshold as a result of many years of academic failure and takes into account the low self-image of these learners. A further aim of the intervention programme is to reduce the impact of these difficulties.

The intervention approach, based on an interdisciplinary theoretical model (Goldfus, 2001), draws on neuroscience and assumes that there are at least two levels in brain consciousness: a cognitive level and a metacognitive level. The metacognitive level controls and monitors the cognitive level (Nelson & Narens, 1994; Schwartz & Perfect, 2002).

> Metacognitive monitoring is those processes that allow the individual to observe, reflect on, or experience his or her own cognitive processes.... Metacognitive control is the conscious and non-conscious decisions that we make based on the output of our monitoring processes. (Schwartz & Perfect, 2002: 4)

By altering the neurological control processes through new learning, it may be possible to improve cognitive learning (Schwartz & Perfect, 2002; Sodian & Frith, 2008).

In the next part, I discuss the conceptual foundations of this intervention programme. It addresses the complexity of both learning disabilities and reading comprehension as a requirement for academic and social success.

Theoretical Framework for the Intervention Programme

The Intervention Programme for students in Secondary School (IPSS) draws on the principles of Wong's Instructional Model (Wong, 1988) for intervention research in learning disabilities. In addition, it operationalises aspects of Gernsbacher's Mental Model (1990) and Bernhardt's Socio-Cognitive Model (1993). The IP is specifically constructed for reading comprehension in English as a foreign language (EFL), in order to enable the learner to read academic texts fluently. Its aim is to break the cycle of failure so that the unsuccessful student can become successful and function at the same level as the regular student.

Wong's (1988) model has three key goals for intervention with learning-disabled (LD) students. The first is to inculcate declarative knowledge (what), procedural knowledge (how) and metacognitive knowledge (monitoring). The second goal is to improve cognitive processing through training activities. The third goal addresses the student's motivation to learn.

According to Wong, declarative knowledge is both conceptual and factual knowledge – 'knowing that'. Declarative knowledge is related to the theoretical notion of schema and text structure, which is modified as a function of incoming information. Procedural knowledge, according to Wong, is 'knowing how'. She argues that successful learning is not only what is known but how new information is integrated. Based on Brown (1980), she argues that successful learning is mediated through an individual's metacognition. She emphasises the minimum four factors to be taken into account in a learning situation: characteristics of the learner, criterial task, that is, learning the goals of the task, learning activities, and the structure of the materials to be learnt.

The second component of her model comprises cognitive processes in learning. These mental operations include students attending to and coding information, rehearsing information or 'chunking' related pieces of information (Wong, 1986: 8). Wong (after Torgesen, 1977) argues that LD students, because of a history of academic failure, have low motivation to learn. Because of the particular nature of LD students' failure-related motivational problems, it may be necessary to build into an intervention a special focus on enhancing motivation to learn, while simultaneously teaching them requisite knowledge (Wong, 1986: 10). She maintains that when LD students understand the nature of their learning problems as they arise and solve them effectively they develop metacognitive knowledge about themselves as learners and about their learning process.

I share Wong's view that intervention is far more complex than simply giving the LD reader strategies and skills and relating the skills to learning. The phenomenon of dyslexia and the difficulty in processing information across modes are very complex and there are no easy solutions. Intervention should be equally complex and should contain many elements, relating to this complexity. Wong raises the point that most intervention programmes train students in strategies and skills. She maintains that this approach bypasses the fundamental reason why these individuals have difficulties in learning despite adequate intelligence and ample opportunity to learn. Wong's criticism of intervention research and current reviews of intervention research in L1 (Foorman & Al Otaiba, 2009; McGill-Franzen & Allington, 2011) concerns the fact that short-term benefits are emphasised and, in recent years, that the focus has been on prevention. Most research on learners of the English language concentrates on RTI (Response to Intervention) – at the level of the kindergarten learner (Siegel, 2009). Wong proposes a conceptual framework so that the intervention will achieve long-term benefits. These principles have been adapted to English as a foreign language (EFL) in the intervention programme presented here, and related to the complexity of skilled reading comprehension, on the one hand, and dyslexia, on the other.

Intervention begins in the mother tongue with the development of 'self' as a prerequisite for cognitive intervention (Goldfus, 2012). Self-awareness and self-efficacy are addressed. The pupils thus learn to understand what it means to have dyslexia or a language-related disability and to develop an awareness of intraindividual versus interindividual achievement (Butler, 1998). In other words, the intervention programme helps the learners understand themselves as learners, with their strengths and difficulties, and to put themselves rather than the teacher at the centre of the learning situation.

Intervention Programme (IPSS)

In this section I present first the basic principles for planning and implementing any intervention programme that will meet the needs of the individual student or group of students with reading comprehension difficulties in L2 or EFL. In developing an intervention programme, specific aims and objectives must be defined (Dockrell & McShane, 1993), and the programme steps then sequenced. To promote efficient learning, material is presented in a way that engages learners' prior knowledge and ensures that each step is linked to the previous one. Organising new information is essential to enable the reader to understand novel material more quickly and thoroughly. The first steps in an intervention programme should be sufficiently easy for learners to gain success at the first attempt, and these early items should be drawn from relevant material.

Not every step or item in an intervention programme is essential for every student; conversely, certain activities may need to be repeated. By repeating a process, automaticity may be achieved, which helps the student to learn information effectively (Stanovich, 1990). Reading comprehension is a complex cognitive process and being able to identify the main idea in text requires much practice. This ability lies at the heart of effective reading. It is also a key area of difficulty for students with dyslexia who have information processing problems.

Students who insist on doing word-for-word translation rarely make much progress in language learning (Bernhardt, 1993). In discussing the unsuccessful foreign language learner, Stern notes that

[the] learner's language does not develop into a well ordered system or network. It remains an untidy assemblage of separate items. He makes no attempt to relate items to each other. Because his approach is passive, unsystematic and fragmented, he will complain that he has no memory for language. (Stern, 1975: 314)

The goal of the programme is to change the individual's passive attitude to active involvement, through a variety of activities which address the areas of difficulty. The expected outcomes are higher motivation and improved reading comprehension and language proficiency in the additional/foreign language.

Motivation

A key feature of the IPSS is developing motivation and self-image in learners who have a history of failure in school reading and learning. The first stage of the IPSS begins with the students' self-assessment of motivation, using a scale of five categories of 'control' (Figure 3.1), from hopefulness or despair (lack of control) to success (taking control). The scale, which is a part of the metacognitive aspect in the theoretical model, promotes the self-image of the students and their gradual development from passive students to those involved and willing to make an effort in their studies. Self-control and self-regulation are developed both through changing their emotions as well as their involvement in the learning situation (intrapersonal). Being able to cope with the academic situation, which previously had caused so much fear and despair, enables them to take responsibility for their learning and to begin to understand how they fit into the learning situation (interpersonal). Once students internalise a positive self-image, learn to assess whether they have understood the text or not, and are able to monitor where they stand with regard to the material to be learned, their sense of self-efficacy translates into self-statements such as 'I can do it'. Control of the situation enables them to move on to the next stage, where cognitive intervention in reading comprehension can take place.

The categories are discussed with the students in their L1. The first two categories 'despair' and 'alienation', legitimise their feelings of failure. They choose from given sentences that match their feeling at that particular time. They also add their own if they feel that their feelings are not adequately

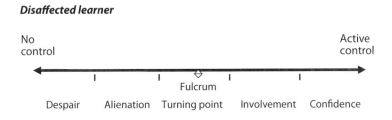

Figure 3.1 Continuum of self-assessment

expressed. The self-assessment is completed at regular intervals through-out the programme. By developing metacognitive awareness, students can change from disaffected learners to active participants in the learning situation. Combined with an acceptance of oneself and one's limitations, a positive attitude can develop to provide motivation for successful academic achievement (Schneider, 2008).

The ability to self-regulate learning and motivation emerges gradually; as passive learners become personally involved in their learning situation, their frustration threshold rises and the desire to quit weakens. Students learn self-control, which is 'critical for success in school' (Sodian & Frith, 2008: 111).

Torgesen (2004) maintains that many students who have dyslexia and who have a history of failure in the classroom have lost their intrinsic motivation to learn. Intrinsic motivation refers to interest in the activity itself, which drives our willingness to exert effort (Alexander *et al.*, 1998). However, when these students succeed, they attribute success to external agents such as luck or teacher behaviour; when they fail, they attribute failure to poor ability. They also have low expectations for success at school (Ellis & Larkin, 1998). Because of the particular nature of these students' failure-related motivational problems, it is necessary to focus on enhancing motivation to learn while simultaneously teaching them reading compre-hension in English as a foreign language. Self-assessment is one way of coming to grips with understanding success and failure.

Understanding (and concentrating on whatever is understood) and being able to point out difficulties are the main aims of the intervention programme. The students are made aware of themselves as learners, of the task that is demanded of them and of the cognitive aspects of that task, so that they are able to understand where their difficulties arise. They gain self-confidence by understanding that it is acceptable to have problems; lack of success does not necessarily mean that they have no value as a person (van Ryzin, 2011). Through teaching literacy skills, declarative and procedural knowledge are cumulative. By repeating the same processes in every text, success and enhanced motivation are gradually achieved .

Successful learning involves the conscious effort of the students. Motiva-tion can come about only if the student is involved in the learning situation. The IP demands the involvement of students and leads them to success. Success provides the motivation needed to continue to succeed.

Intervention for reading comprehension

The IPSS approaches reading comprehension intersententially and intrasententially. The aim is not only to provide strategies, but to intervene cognitively so that the reader learns to process information and read success-fully in English as a foreign language. By developing the ability to construct the main idea, disregarding information which is not necessary, the student with difficulties in learning reading comprehension is led along the path to success.

> the notion of reading strategies may be applicable at many levels of comprehension processing and its functioning in cognitive processing accounts of reading is not clear.... There needs to be a greater effort to incorporate these issues into the cognitive processing research on reading comprehension. There needs to be much more research on the various types of strategies that are used, when they are used, how they are used, why they are used, who uses them and in what combinations they are used. (Grabe, 2000: 23)

The aim of the IPSS is to help the at-risk reader to process information rather than only read words, and to achieve an outcome similar to that of a skilled reader. There is a tendency in pedagogy in general, and 'remedial' teaching in particular, to infantilise learners and to maintain them in a state of intellectual and emotional dependency on teachers, course materials and tightly organised 'methods'. Cognitive intervention is seen as 'cognitive rehabilitation', where, rather than focusing on poor language skills and vocabulary, the older learner is given credit for sophisticated ideas. The IPSS is based on the assumption that processing abilities develop over time. This presupposes that learning is not linear, that is, one element is not simply replaced by another, but the process is interactive, global and multi-dimensional. At the reading comprehension level (i.e. the cognitive level), emphasis is placed forming a coherent understanding of the expository text (Gernsbacher, 1990). On the macro-level, the students are shown how to organise passage content into main ideas and sub-ideas (Bernhardt, 1993). On the micro-level, training focuses on the understanding of anaphoric relations, connectives and reference in order to establish cohesion within sentences.

Students are taught to find connections between words, to understand the grammar of a sentence (intrasentential) and between sentences (intersentential) so that they understand the meaning within and across sentences. The main idea is written (or spoken) in the learner's mother tongue. First, the readers are taught to notice, judge and be able to decide what is important and what is not. The teacher's questions guide the reader in being able to reconstruct a text that has meaning. This inter-action develops the procedural knowledge (how). The method remains the same across different texts, so that automaticity is achieved, although the texts become longer, and more complex grammar and new vocabulary are introduced. By way of example, four exercises of the IPSS are presented in Figure 3.2.

Read the passage.

Headbands

The headband was popular in ancient times. They were worn again by women in the 1920s and again by hippies in the 1960s and by tennis-players in the 1990s.

Exercise 1:

Who wore the headbands?

a. Who: _____   _____   _____
b. When: _____   _____   _____

What is the main idea? [One or two sentences in L1.]

Read the passage and pay attention to the words that 'stand' for: *denim* and *Levi Strauss*.

Jeans

In America in the 1850s, men working in the gold mines wore trousers made of canvas. In the 1860s a man named Levi Strauss used a softer material called denim. Then this clever man dyed the light coloured fabric blue. He did this to hide the stains as much as possible. As an extra touch, the genius added a lot of pockets so that the miners would be able to carry all their tools comfortably. The main idea is _____

Exercise 2:

List words that stand for:

a. denim   _____
b. Levi Strauss _____

Read the next paragraph and this time pay attention to the pronouns: *they* and *them*.

Cowboys

Cowboys liked the new pants but [1]they wanted [2]them to fit very tightly. So [3]they put [4]them on, got into a tub of hot water and then lay in the sun until [5]they dried. The denims shrank in the sun and fitted each cowboy perfectly. [6]They were able to ride their horses more comfortably. Jeans became very popular.

Exercise 3:

Who or what does each *they* and *them* stand for.
Write the numbers in the appropriate column.

	they	*them*
The cowboys		
The pants		

Exercise 4:

Find 3 places where you can add *they*. Fill them in.
Cowboys liked the new pants but they wanted them to fit very tightly. So they put them on, got into a tub of hot water and then lay in the sun until they dried. The denims shrank in the sun and fitted each cowboy perfectly. They were able to ride their horses more comfortably. Jeans became very popular.

Figure 3.2 Four example exercises from the intervention programme. In the passage called 'Cowboys' the distinction between subject and object is highlighted so that an awareness of grammatical ambiguity and deletion to avoid repetition is taught. In 'Cowboys' the area that is taught is to differentiate between the words 'they' and 'them', subject and object

Grammar and word order are important elements in comprehension. Adams (1980) comments that grammar (syntax) is the primary means by which we can specify the intended relation between words:

> If readers cannot recognize a word, they generally know they cannot. If they cannot correctly recognize a syntactic structure, they may not even realize it. Further, at the lexical level, it is easy to distinguish between where the readers do not know a word or just cannot read it. The parallel distinction at the syntactic level may be unclear. (Adams, 1980: 23)

In teaching, grammar is rarely viewed in its functional sense, that is, as indicating intrasentential connections. In the learning situation, 'grammar' as sentence structure is kept conceptually distinct from semantics, that is, meaning. An inability to understand grammar and word order leads to a breakdown in the reading process or, in many cases, to an incorrect interpretation of the text. If the grammatical relationship between the words is not understood and the initial comprehension is erroneous, a coherent understanding of the text cannot be achieved.

It is through difficulties and errors that assessments can be made of whether a specific intervention is needed or not. For example, in 'Cowboys' (Figure 3.2) one student wrote that the main idea was that 'the cowboys wanted faded jeans'. By understanding how he came to this conclusion, I realised that he thought the word 'tightly' was 'lighter'. Not only did he not understand the part of speech, that 'ly' denotes an adverb, but he had read 'l' for 't' and connected it with the word 'sun' and come up with 'faded'.

Text structure

Fundamental to the interactive view of reading is the fact that comprehension results from the joint construction of meaning between the author of the text and the reader. The term 'text structure' is used to refer to the way ideas in a text are interrelated to convey a message. Comprehension breaks down when there is an inability to find the connection between the referent and the relevant part in previous information. The IPSS aims to increase the learner's ability to make connections across sentences so that the emphasis is on meaning and coherence, leading to a continuous growth of an understanding of how reading and literacy skills work. To sum up, misunderstandings can be traced to the learner's inability to extract the main idea and sub-ideas, to flawed understanding of grammar and grammatical relationships between words, as well as to lexical difficulties. Figure 3.3 presents a further example. Such exercises emphasise the importance of connecting ideas and being able to construct the overall meaning (Garrod & Sanford, 1994). The example in Figure 3.3 illustrates how relative pronouns sequence a passage logically. The learner is taught to recognise the

A girl wanted to buy a book for a friend. She went to a bookstore and chose a title that she liked. But she had forgotten to take her glasses with her so she couldn't read the text on the back cover. However, she bought it and then went home, put on her glasses and read the text. Of course, the book was totally unsuitable. She immediately phoned the bookstore and asked if she could change it. Luckily they agreed.

Underline the **connectors** and **pronouns**.

Write this _____ for pronouns.

Write this _ _ _ _ _ _ _ _ _ for connectors

What is the main idea? [One or two sentences in L1.]

Figure 3.3 Example exercise from the intervention programme dealing with text structure

importance of connectors, which are the markers of cohesion, and pronouns, as contributing to coherence. On a metacognitive level, the aim of these units is to create an awareness of connectors and pronouns, to understand the connections of ideas and to be able then to add or change the cognitive schema, and to understand the information accordingly.

It is assumed that the at-risk learner has had these structures explained many times, as the relative pronoun appears in all the grammar books. The use of anaphoric relations and relative pronouns to link ideas from adjacent sentences are viewed as essential and integral to comprehension. However, understanding the meaning of sentences where the relative pronoun or clause appears still proves to be problematic. Students are unable to find the connection and thus a breakdown in comprehension occurs. By introducing this very problematic area in another way, it is hoped that students are engaged in processing the information differently, so that when they come across this structure in other texts they are able to comprehend the text successfully. That is, they 'transfer' or expand the conceptual remit of their learning to include similar examples of the grammatical structures and are able to understand the new text.

Emphasis is placed on coherence and the ability to find the connections between sentences and to construct a mental model. The questions (who, what, where, when) indicate tasks which always relate to the referential texture of a particular text. In this way, students are guided to understand how to process information by focusing on a particular feature. The aim is to develop an awareness of the processes involved in reading comprehension, so that a conscious effort is expended to learn the instructed concept, to practise it to mastery (automaticity) and to maintain and generalise its use beyond the original context (Paris *et al.*, 1994).

Intervention provides the at-risk learner with the ability to engage with the learning situation, to succeed and hence become motivated in an iterative cycle. The IPSS attempts to lower the stress level that is associated with English as a foreign language. This approach relates to adolescents with respect to and with regard for their sophistication in a complex world. One of the comments frequently made by adolescents with dyslexia is 'I know it and understand it in my head, but when I write it or say it, it does not come out correctly and I fail.' The IPSS, as an intervention tool, provides 'scaffolding' for this group of learners, so that they are able to express what they understand.

The IPSS and the Role of Teachers

The efficacy of the IPSS depends on teachers' understanding of severe difficulties in reading comprehension, and their knowledge and ability to involve the student in the act of learning. Within the social setting of the classroom, the teacher must be aware of the student as a learner, since the aim of effective teaching is not to teach the material, but to teach the student. Developing learners' positive attitude and motivation towards the learning process are important factors in successful teaching. The approach discussed here provides scaffolding to support this group of learners. When the reader has success and understands the passages, a positive response is generated, cognitive intervention can begin and the gap between the regular learner and the learner with dyslexia narrows. In other words, the teacher must provide explanations which are clear, well structured and organised so that intervention can help the students (Reid, 1998; Stone, 1998; Wharton-McDonald, 2011).

When asked what a paragraph is about, a good portion of students with a learning disability cannot provide the general topic. The ability of the teacher to ask the right questions and 'scaffold' instruction is a very important skill in teaching the at-risk learner. The aim of the questions is to promote attention to the connective devices and to lead the students to connect ideas and construct the main idea. Having identified the main idea, the students then circle reference to the general topic in each sentence in the paragraph. The teacher, in this situation, becomes the facilitator and encourages the students to 'work with the texts'. Understanding and constructing the main idea is an appropriate beginning in the development of a complex fundamental comprehension process. Most remedial instructional programmes in EFL reading are oriented towards beginning reading and decoding (Gunderson & D'Silva, 2011). When texts increase in difficulty, the IP approach and steps used in processing information remain consistent.

Conclusions

Skilled learners command a large body of conceptual and procedural knowledge. Their rich declarative and procedural knowledge facilitates new learning because new information can be related readily to prior knowledge. This is how cognitive intervention should operate. On the one hand, it increases declarative knowledge by providing articles about different subjects so that the schemata of the students with learning disabilities can be developed (Stanovich, 1986; Stanovich et al., 1996). On the other hand, procedural knowledge is developed by focusing on the 'how', through the various questions and by repeating the same process so that 'automaticity' is achieved. In this way, students are able to 'map' information rather than to 'shift' it. In addition, metacognitive knowledge is emphasised because it permits clarity of learning goals, teaches self-monitoring, leads to a positive self-image and enables the dysfunctional student to cope with the academic situation. If IPSS requires the learning-disabled student to combine declarative knowledge, procedural knowledge and metacognitive knowledge; as such, the three become one focus for the learning-disabled student. This merger is the essence of the proposed IPSS.

The IPSS operationalises the principles of several cognitive models, namely Wong's Instructional Model (1988), Gernsbacher's Mental Model (1990) and Bernhardt's Socio-Cognitive Model (1993). Further, the development of learners' metacognitive awareness has been illustrated and discussed in depth. The role of the teachers in the IPSS is mentioned throughout although, as the chapter deals with reading comprehension from the point of view of the reader's learning, teaching is not discussed in as much detail. It is obvious that intervention cannot take place successfully without high-quality teaching.

The work presented in this chapter has examined severe reading comprehension difficulties in the contexts of English as an additional or foreign language, through a cognitive psychology lens, which is the dominant paradigm in dyslexia research. It contributes to the body of knowledge of dyslexia in a number of important ways. It offers a focus on intervention rather than on the more familiar research site of identification of reading difficulties. It examines reading comprehension of older learners and discusses the unique difficulties that they bring to teaching and learning literacy skills. The chapter discusses an under-researched yet increasingly important site of research and pedagogy, that of dyslexia and difficulties in acquiring literacy skills in contexts of English as an additional or foreign language. Further research could examine how intervention could be implemented with bilingual speakers of other additional or foreign languages.

References

Adams, M.J. (1980) Failures to comprehend and levels of processing in reading. In R.J. Spiro, B.B. Bruce and W.F. Brewer (eds) *Theoretical Issues in Reading Comprehension* (pp. 11–32). Hillsdale, NJ: Erlbaum.

Alexander, P.A., Garner, R., Sperl, C.T. and Hare, V.C. (1998) Fostering reading competence in students with learning disabilities. In B.Y.L. Wong (ed.) *Learning About Learning Disabilities* (pp. 343–366). London: Academic Press.

Bernhardt, E.B. (1993) *Reading Development in a Second Language: Theoretical, Empirical and Classroom Perspectives* (2nd edn). Norwood, NJ: Ablex Publishing.

Brown, A.L. (1980) Metacognitive development and reading. In R.J. Spiro, B.B. Bruce and W.F. Brewer (eds) *Theoretical Issues in Reading Comprehension* (pp. 11–32). Hillsdale, NJ: Erlbaum.

Butler, D. (1998) Metacognition and learning disabilities. In B. Wong (ed.) *Learning About Learning Disabilities* (pp. 277–303). New York: Elsevier Academic Press.

Cutting, L.E., Eason, S.H., Young, D.M. and Alberstadt, A.L. (2009) Reading comprehension: Cognition and neuroimaging. In K. Pugh and P. McCardle (eds) *How Children Learn to Read* (pp. 195–209). Abingdon: Psychology Press.

Dockrell, J. and McShane, J. (1993) *Children's Learning Difficulties: A Cognitive Approach*. Oxford: Blackwell.

Ehrlich, M-F. (1996) Metacognitive monitoring in the processing of anaphoric devices in skilled and less skilled comprehenders. In C.Cornoldi and J.Oakhill (eds) *Reading Comprehension Difficulties: Processes and Intervention* (pp. 221–249). Mahwah, NJ: Lawrence Erlbaum.

Ellis, E.S. and Larkin, M.J. (1998) Strategic instruction for adolescents with learning disabilities. In B.Y.L. Wong (ed.) *Learning About Learning Disabilities* (pp. 585–656). London: Academic Press.

Flavell, J.H. (1976) Metacognitive aspects of problem solving. In L.B. Resnick (ed.) *The Nature of Intelligence* (pp. 231–236). Hillsdale, NJ: Erlbaum.

Foorman, B. and Al Otaiba, A. (2009) Reading remediation: State of the art. In K. Pugh and P. McCardle (eds) *How Children Learn to Read* (pp. 257–274). Abingdon: Psychology Press.

Ganschow, L., Sparks, R.L. and Javorsky, J. (1998) Foreign language learning difficulties: An historical perspective. *Journal of Learning Disabilities* 31(3), 248–258.

Garner, R. (1987) *Metacognition and Reading Comprehension*. Norwood, NJ: Ablex Publishing.

Garrod, S.C. and Sanford, A.J. (1994) Resolving sentences in a discourse context. How discourse representation affects language understanding. *Handbook of Psycholinguistics* (pp. 675–698). New York: Academic Press.

Gernsbacher, M.A. (1990) *Language Comprehension as Structure Building*. Hillsdale, NJ: Erlbaum.

Ghelani, K., Sidhu, R., Jain, U. and Tannock, R. (2004) Reading comprehension and reading related abilities in adolescents with reading disabilities and attention-deficit/hyperactivity disorder. *Dyslexia* 10, 364–384.

Goldfus, C.I. (2001) Reading comprehension and EFL adolescents with difficulties: a cognitive processing model. Unpublished doctoral thesis, University of Birmingham.

Goldfus, C.I. (2010) Is there a connection between reading disabilities and a general automaticity deficit? Paper presented at the international conference of the International Academy for Research in Learning Disabilities (IARLD), Miami, Florida.

Goldfus, C.I. (2012) Intervention through metacognitive development: A case study of a student with dyslexia and comorbid attention deficit disorder. *Journal of Language and Culture*, 3 (3), 56–66. DOI: 10.5897/JLC11.042.

Grabe, W. (2000) Developments in reading research and their implications for computer-adaptive reading assessment. In M. Chalhoub-Deville (ed.) *Issues in Computer Adaptive Testing of Reading Proficiency* (pp. 11–47). Cambridge: Cambridge University Press.

Grabe, W. (2009) *Reading in a Second Language: Moving from Theory to Practice.* New York: Cambridge University Press.

Gunderson, L. and D'Silva, R. (2011) Second language reading disability: International themes. In A. McGill-Franzen and R.L. Allington (eds) *Handbook of Reading Disability Research* (pp. 13–24). New York: Routledge, Taylor and Francis.

Kintsch, W. and Rawson, K.A. (2005) Comprehension. In M.J. Snowling and C. Hulme (eds) *The Science of Reading: A Handbook* (pp. 209–226). Oxford: Blackwell.

Koda, K. (2005) *Insights Into Second Language Reading. A Cross-linguistic Approach.* Cambridge: Cambridge University Press.

Mayer, R.E. (2008) Multimedia literacy. In J. Coiro, M. Knobel, C. Lankshear and D. Leu (eds) *Handbook of Research on New Literacies* (pp. 359–376). London: Taylor and Francis.

McGill-Franzen, A. and Allington, R.L. (2011) *Handbook of Reading Disability Research.* New York: Routledge, Taylor and Francis.

Nelson, T.O. and Narens, L. (1994) Why investigate metacognition? In J. Metcalfe and A.P. Shimamura (eds) *Metacognition: Knowing About Knowing* (pp. 1–25). The MIT Press, Cambridge, MA.

Nicolson, R. I. and Fawcett, A.J. (2008). *Dyslexia, Learning, and the Brain.* Cambridge, MA: MIT Press.

Oakhill, J. and Garnham, A. (1988) *Becoming a Skilled Reader.* Oxford: Blackwell.

Oakhill, J. and Yuill, N. (1996) Higher order factors in comprehension disability: Processes and remediation. In C. Cornoldi and J. Oakhill (eds) *Reading Comprehension Difficulties: Processes and Intervention* (pp. 69–92). Hillsdale, NJ: Erlbaum.

Paris, S.G., Lipson, M.Y., and Wixson, K.K. (1994) Becoming a strategic reader. In R.B. Ruddell, M.R. Ruddell and H. Singer (eds) *Theoretical Models and Processes of Reading* (4th edn) (pp. 788–811). Newark, DE: International Reading Association.

Perfetti, C.A. (1994) Psycholinguistics and reading ability. In M.A. Gernsbacher (ed.) *Handbook of Psycholinguistics* (pp. 849–894). San Diego, CA: Academic Press.

Perfetti, C.A., Marron, M.A. and Foltz, P.W. (1996) Sources of comprehension failure: Theoretical perspectives and case studies. In C. Cornoldi and J. Oakhill (eds) *Reading Comprehension Difficulties: Processes and Intervention* (pp. 137–165). Hillsdale, NJ: Erlbaum.

Perfetti, C.A., Landi, N. and Oakhill, J. (2005) The acquisition of reading comprehension skill. In M.J. Snowling and C. Hulme (eds) *The Science of Reading: A Handbook* (pp. 227–247). Oxford: Blackwell.

Randall, M. (2007) *Memory, Psychology and Second Language Learning.* Amsterdam: John Benjamins Publishing.

Reid, D.K. (1998) Scaffolding: A broader view. *Journal of Learning Disabilities* 33 (4), 386–396.

Schmalhofer, F. and Perfetti, C.A. (2007) Neural behavioral indicators of integration processes across sentence boundaries. In C.A. Perfetti and F. Schmalhofer (eds) *Higher Level Language Processes in the Brain* (pp. 161–188). Mahwah, NJ: Lawrence Erlbaum.

Schneider, W. (2008) The development of metacognitive knowledge in children and adolescents: Major trends and implications for education. *Mind, Brain and Education* 2, 114–121.

Schwartz, B.L. and Perfect, T.J. (2002) Introduction: Toward an applied metacognition. In T.J. Perfect and B.L. Schwartz (eds) *Applied Metacognition* (pp. 1–11). Cambridge: Cambridge University Press.

Shaywitz, S. (2003) *Overcoming Dyslexia.* New York: Alfred A. Knopf.

Siegel, L.S. (2009) Remediation of reading difficulties in English-language learning students. In K. Pugh and P. McCardle (eds) *How Children Learn to Read* (pp. 275–288). Abindon: Psychology Press.

Sodian, B. and Frith, U. (2008) Metacognition, theory of mind, and self-control: The relevance of high-level cognitive processes in development, neuroscience, and education. *Mind, Brain and Education* 2, 111–113.

Sparks, R.L., Schneider, E. and Ganschow, L. (2002) Teaching foreign (second) language to at-risk learners: Research and practice. In J-A. Hammadou Sullivan (ed.) *Literacy and the Second Language Learner* (pp. 55–84). Charlotte, NC: Information Age Publishing.

Sparks, R., Patton, J., Ganschow, L. and Humbach, N. (2009) Long-term cross-linguistic transfer of skills from L1 to L2. *Language Learning* 59 (1), 203–243.

Stanovich, K.E. (1986) Matthew effects in reading: Some consequences of individual differences in the acquisition of literacy. *Reading Research Quarterly* 21, 360–407.

Stanovich, K.E. (1990) Concepts of developmental theories of reading skill: Cognitive resources, automaticity, and modularity. *Developmental Review* 10, 72–100.

Stanovich, K.E., West, R.F., Cunningham, A.E., Cipielewski, J. and Siddiqui, S. (1996) The role of inadequate print exposure as a determinant of reading comprehension problems. In C. Conoldi and J. Oakhill (eds) *Reading Comprehension Difficulties: Processes and Intervention* (pp. 15–32). Hillsdale, NJ: Erlbaum.

Stern, H.H. (1975) What can we learn from the good language learner? *Canadian Modern Language Review* 31, 304–318.

Stone, C.A. (1998) The metaphor of scaffolding: Its utility for the field of learning disabilities. *Journal of Learning Disabilities* 33 (4), 344–364.

Torgesen, J.K. (1977) The role of non-specific factors in the task performance of learning disabled children: A theoretical assessment. *Journal of Learning Disabilities* 10, 27–34.

Torgesen, J.K. (2004) Learning disabilities: An overview. In B. Wong (ed.) *Learning About Learning Disabilities* (pp. 20–25). New York: Elsevier Academic Press.

van Ryzin, M.J. (2011) Motivation and reading disabilities. In A. McGill-Franzen and R.L. Allington (eds) *Handbook of Reading Disability Research* (pp. 242–252). New York: Routledge, Taylor and Francis.

Vellutino, F.R. and Fletcher, J.M. (2005) Developmental dyslexia. In M.J. Snowling and C. Hulme (eds) *The Science of Reading: A Handbook* (pp. 362–378). Oxford: Blackwell.

Westby, C. (2002) Beyond decoding: Critical and dynamic literacy for students with dyslexia, language learning disabilities (LLD), or attention deficit-hyperactivity disorder (ADHD). In K.G. Butler and E.R. Silliman (eds) *Speaking, Reading, and Writing in Children with Language Learning Disabilities* (pp. 73–108). Hillsdale, NJ: Erlbaum.

Wharton-McDonald, R. (2011) Expert classroom instruction for students with reading disabilities: Explicit, intense, targeted … and flexible. In A. McGill-Franzen and R.L. Allington (eds) *Handbook of Reading Disability Research* (pp. 265–272). New York: Routledge, Taylor and Francis.

Wong, B.Y.L. (1986) Metacognition and special education: A review of a view. *Journal of Special Education* 20, 9–29.

Wong, B.Y.L. (1988) An instructional model for intervention research in learning disabilities. *Learning Disabilities Research* 4 (1), 5–16.

Yuill, N. and Oakhill, J. (1991) *Children's Problems in Text Comprehension: An Experimental Investigation.* Cambridge: Cambridge University Press.

4 Assessing Research on Dyslexic Language Learners in Contexts With English as a Foreign Language

Judit Kormos

Introduction

This chapter reviews research conducted on dyslexic language learners in the context of English as a foreign language (EFL). In many countries, proficiency in English is often as important as other basic competencies such as literacy and arithmetic skills. Nevertheless, students who have specific learning differences (SpLDs) rarely receive assistance with language learning, due to the assumption that they cannot be expected to acquire a second language (L2) successfully because of the literacy-related difficulties they experience in their native language. To counter this widely held belief in the field of educational policy and to ensure that multilingualism is an attainable goal for everyone, current research on the foreign language learning processes of students with SpLDs, more specifically those with dyslexia, has been directed at understanding the foreign language learning difficulties and mechanisms of those learners and discovering what instructional practices are effective in teaching them.

This chapter focuses on studies conducted on dyslexic language learners in European countries, where English is taught as a foreign language in classroom settings. In most of these studies, dyslexia is seen as an SpLD, one which has neurological origins, and is often treated as an individual difference variable, similar to language aptitude, that affects learning processes and performance in the classroom and in standardised language tests. Consequently, most studies are conducted in relation to biological and medical models of disability, and many of them adopt an etic perspective, in which the researcher remains an outsider in the research context. The focus of research in this field has mostly been on the individual learner and the effectiveness of instructional programmes specifically designed for students with SpLDs. Studies conducted in this paradigm have mainly used survey instruments and language tests that are administered to dyslexic and non-dyslexic students to compare their disposition to learning – for example motivation (Kormos & Csizér, 2010) and anxiety (Piechurska-Kuciel, 2008) – and language performance (e.g. Helland & Kaasa, 2005). The characteristics of dyslexic and non-dyslexic students are contrasted and the former group's differences with the latter learners are often seen as impairments and deficiencies. Research that aims to present the processes of learning EFL from the students' own perspective and which adopts an emic perspective is scarce. Furthermore, studies that view language learners with SpLDs as a diverse group interdependent with the social and instructional context are rare and primarily rely on interview data (e.g. Csizér *et al.*, 2010; Kormos *et al.*, 2009). The barriers present in current foreign language teaching practices and educational policies have remained largely uninvestigated.

This chapter proceeds with an overview of the key concepts of dyslexia and multilingualism in EFL research and shows how these constructs are defined in the biological–medical models that are prevalent in studies on SpLDs and foreign language learning. This is followed by a detailed discussion of how quantitative and qualitative research methods are used in investigations of language learners with SpLDs and how they reflect views of SpLDs, bilingualism and learning. The chapter concludes with recommendations for further research in this field.

Key Concepts of and Assumptions About Dyslexia and Multilingualism in Research on the Acquisition of a Foreign Language

The way language is used to describe learning difficulties reflects how society perceives their characteristics and effect on learning and also shapes how teachers and researchers relate to students who display a different approach to learning. For example, the definition of 'disability' in the British Disability Discrimination Act 1995 states that disability is 'a physical or mental impairment which has a substantial and long-term adverse effect on the ability to carry out normal day-to-day activities' (Department of Trade and Industry, 1995). This definition implies that disability constitutes a series of barriers in students' lives and that students with disability show deficiencies when compared with others. This view, which exemplifies biological–medical models of SpLDs, suggests that the source of the problem is the individual and that the responsibility of the scientific community and education is to find the cause of the problem and offer a treatment for it. In this model, students are seen as having individual needs that have to be met by special education providers, schools and other institutions of education. In contrast, the view of SpLDs as a socially constructed barrier, which is also expressed by the United Nations Convention on the Rights of Persons with Disabilities (2006), sees disabled people as those 'who have long-term physical, mental, intellectual or sensory impairments which in interaction with various barriers may hinder their full and effective participation in society on an equal basis with others' (United Nations, 2006: 4). This model places the emphasis on disabling factors in society and the environment, rather than locating any difficulties in the individual (Ahmad, 2000). Unfortunately, this sociocultural model of disability is rarely referred to in studies in the field of foreign language learning.

One of the reasons for the prevalence of the biological–medical model of disabilities in researching dyslexia in foreign language contexts is that most studies to date have been conducted in the psycholinguistic paradigm, which regards language learning as a cognitive process. Many studies on the role of dyslexia in language learning (e.g. Helland, 2008; Helland & Kaasa, 2005; Nijakowska, 2008, 2010) see foreign language learning as the acquisition of linguistic skills, including speaking, writing, listening and reading, and focus on individual language learners, isolating them from the environment in which learning takes place. Researchers in this field tend to adopt an information-processing view of language learning, according to which students receive input, process it and then produce some kind of output and apply cognitive strategies to aid their learning processes (e.g. Downey et al., 2000). Language learners are assumed to display different cognitive and affective individual characteristics, such as motivation, language learning anxiety and aptitude (Kormos & Csizér, 2010; Piechurska-Kuciel, 2008), which are regarded as inherent and stable characteristics of learners, independent of context. In these studies, not only are learners seen to be separate from their environment, but language is also viewed as an abstract and isolated entity, which is mainly used within the boundaries of the classroom and not as a tool for social interaction.

Bilingualism in this paradigm is regarded as knowledge of a foreign language which is additional to the student's mother tongue. In EFL contexts, English is acquired in instructional settings, and in many European countries students in the public school system rarely use English outside the classroom. In many contexts, however, especially after students leave school, English is considered a lingua franca and plays a mediating role between speakers of different languages. English is the language of technology, business, science, tourism and entertainment. Bilingualism does not necessarily mean that in these situations speakers have a native or near-native proficiency in both languages or that both languages are regularly used for everyday purposes. In foreign language contexts, a bilingual person is someone who can use another language to meet their communication needs in situations where knowledge of another language is required. From this perspective, bilingualism entails linguistic competence: the ability to understand and produce spoken and written language, and sociolinguistic and discourse competences (Canale & Swain, 1980). Research in the field of dyslexia and foreign language learning has mainly focused on the acquisition of such linguistic competence.

Methodological Paradigms in Researching Dyslexia in Foreign Language Contexts

Most research in the field of foreign language learning and dyslexia has been conducted within the positivist paradigm, which is a philosophy of science that made its way into social sciences from the natural sciences. The underlying assumptions of positivism are that we can understand phenomena through empirical observation and that scientific knowledge is objective and can be derived independently of the context in which the observation is made. As a consequence, the researcher is seen as separate from the object of study and takes an outsider's perspective. In this kind of research, hypotheses are set up for a study a priori; they are tested and a large number of observations are made to ensure that findings are generalisable. Studies within this paradigm are quantitative in nature and collect data from a large number of respondents. As figures are generally reported with reference to averages, this type of research offers few insights into individual variation between participants and describes typicality rather than diversity. As Constable (2001) points out, students with SpLDs might exhibit similar behaviour and achieve similar test scores, but their underlying difficulties and the strategies they use to overcome their difficulties might be different, which quantitative studies are not able to account for. The most important research techniques applied within this paradigm are questionnaires and experiments in which a limited set of variables is manipulated in order to establish cause–effect relationships. In linguistic research, large samples of language performance are also analysed to identify general tendencies in language use.

In contrast to the positivist research tradition, social constructivists argue that scientific observations are context dependent and influenced by the views, beliefs and experiences of the observer (for a review see Guba & Lincoln, 1989). In their view, the main aim of research in the social sciences is to provide rich descriptions of phenomena from the perspective of those who are studied so that readers can gain an in-depth understanding of a particular case (Guba & Lincoln, 1989). In this paradigm, interpretations of findings are socially constructed and phenomena are assumed to have multiple interacting causes. This paradigm focuses on the individual and heterogeneity and has the potential to uncover underlying differences in behaviour, attitudes and experience. The research methods used in this framework include interviews, observations, diaries and ethnographic case studies. Considerably fewer studies have been conducted within this methodological paradigm than within the positivist tradition in the field of dyslexia and language learning. In what follows I review and critically analyse the use of different research methods in the field of dyslexia and foreign language learning.

Questionnaires

With regard to foreign language learning and dyslexia, questionnaires have been used to investigate individual differences among dyslexic language learners and to compare the motivational (Kormos & Csizér, 2010) and affective characteristics (Piechurska-Kuciel, 2008) of dyslexic and non-dyslexic students. Motivation, language learning anxiety and self-confidence are generally listed among the most important affective factors that might influence language learning outcomes.

'Motivation explains why people decide to do something, how hard they are going to pursue it and how long they are willing to sustain the activity' (Dörnyei, 2001: 7). The acquisition of a complex skill, such as mastering another language, is hardly possible without sustained effort and persistence as well as clearly stated goals. As a consequence, motivation has a significant effect on attainment in language learning (for a review see Dörnyei, 2005).

Language learning anxiety is usually defined as 'a distinct complex of self-perceptions, beliefs, feelings, and behaviours arising from the unique-ness of the language learning process' in the classroom (Horwitz et al., 1986: 128). In other words, language learning anxiety is situation specific and occurs in the context of classroom language learning. Anxiety has signifi-cant effects on cognition. Due to worry and intrusive thoughts, the working memory capacity of anxious students is reduced, which can slow down the processing of input and the production of output, as well as increase the error rate in these processes (Eysenck & Calvo, 1992; MacIntyre & Gardner, 1994; Tobias & Everson, 1997). Anxiety may also hinder the encoding of new information in long-term memory.

Self-confidence may be defined here as one's perception of the chances of succeeding in learning another language. Without a positive appreciation of one's abilities and chances of success, effective learning is unlikely to happen (Bandura, 1986).

Piechurska-Kuciel (2008) administered a questionnaire to investigate anxiety levels in the three stages of language processing – input, process-ing and output – by Polish secondary school students with what she called developmental dyslexia symptoms. Developmental dyslexia symptoms were assessed with the help of a questionnaire: the Revised Adult Dyslexia Checklist (Vinegrad, 1994). Students with developmental dyslexia symptoms exhibited significantly higher levels of anxiety at all stages of language processing than students who reported no dyslexic symptoms. The anxiety experienced by the group with no dyslexia in the input and pro-cessing stages decreased significantly after the first year of secondary school, then remained stable throughout the subsequent two years of secondary education. However, anxiety at the output stage in students with dyslexia symptoms was found to remain permanently high throughout their whole secondary school career.

The innovative nature of this study was that it had a longitudinal design, and hence it was able to show how levels of anxiety change during secondary school years. The findings of the research, however, were mainly interpreted with reference to psychological theories of language processing, and no detailed discussion was offered of how the instructional and social setting might have influenced the development of anxiety. Another problematic aspect of this research concerned the application of a checklist to identify participants with SpLDs, as self-reported literacy-related difficulties may not provide an adequate basis for identification.

In a recent questionnaire survey conducted on Hungarian dyslexic learners of English and German, Kormos and Csizér (2010) found that dyslexic language learners displayed markedly different motivational characteristics from their non-dyslexic peers. Regardless of which language the surveyed Hungarian students studied and whether or not they had an official diagnosis of dyslexia, one of the most important direct predictors of how much effort they were willing to invest in language learning was their image of themselves as language learners. The findings of the study also indicate that language learning experiences and teachers' behaviour and instructional practices affect students' enthusiasm for language learning. Additionally, the dyslexic language learners displayed significantly different motivational characteristics from their non-dyslexic peers, which was apparent in their language learning self-concepts, attitudes and motivation. The authors hypothesised that the relatively low level of motivation of dyslexic students was likely to be caused by their difficulties in language learning and inappropriate instructional practices. They argued that language learners with dyslexia might easily get caught up in a vicious circle; due to their problems in language learning, they might lose their motivation, which might then lead to the experience of further failures. Furthermore, the dyslexic students seemed to receive less support from their parents in language learning than those who had no apparent learning difficulties.

Kormos and Csizér's (2010) study differs from that of Piechurska-Kuciel (2008) in that their dyslexic participants were in possession of an official document certifying their SpLD, whereas Piechurska-Kuciel used a checklist of dyslexia symptoms to identify students with difficulties in acquiring literacy skills. A methodological innovation in Kormos and Csizér's study was that dyslexic primary school students had the questionnaire read out to them, and this had previously been carefully piloted to make sure that the wording was simple and understandable for dyslexic participants. Both questionnaire studies were quantitative in nature; they applied statistical procedures and tests of significance to analyse the data and aimed to be able to generalise their findings to other contexts.

These studies provide important evidence that many students with SpLDs often feel anxious and under-motivated and may have a negative self-concept and low self-confidence in language learning. Furthermore, this kind of research is helpful in describing the affective profile of dyslexic language learners in general. However, the nature of questionnaire research is such that it gives us a view of the hypothetical 'average' student but reveals little about variation among participants. This is particularly problematic in the case of language learners with SpLDs, as they might have very different individual characteristics, strengths and weaknesses. In addition, this line of research exhibits some of the shortcomings of studies conducted in line with the biological–medical view of disability. First, in both projects, the reference group consisted of students who did not seem to demonstrate learning difficulties. It might not be appropriate to consider non-dyslexic students as a basis for comparison, as this assumes that the 'norm' is the way students with no apparent SpLDs feel or behave. Second, although Kormos and Csizér's study made an attempt to investigate the role of immediate social context and instructional practices in motivation and attitudes, neither their study nor that of Piechurska-Kuciel could yield detailed insights into why dyslexic students experience anxiety and what causes their lack of motivation in the contexts investigated.

Experiments

Another type of research in the positivist tradition includes the use of experiments. In an experiment, the researcher usually manipulates one variable in a process called treatment, while keeping all other factors constant, and observes the effect of the change in that variable on different outcome measures. The ultimate aim of experimental research is to demonstrate the existence of causal relations between treatment and dependent variable. In studies in the field of language learning, students in an experiment receive focused instruction on an element of language and their improvement is compared with that of a control group. Although experimental research helps us understand the effect on learning of different instructional conditions and methods, this type of research might lack internal validity because intervening variables are often difficult to control, particularly in classroom settings. Furthermore, experiments in one particular context might not often be generalisable to other instructional and social situations.

An example of an experimental study is the one conducted by Nijakowska (2008), who investigated the effectiveness of direct multisensory instruction for improving word reading and spelling skills in English through the systematic study of selected grapheme–phoneme relations and spelling rules. Three groups of Polish learners of English participated in her study: one experimental and two control groups. The students' progress was measured by a series of reading and spelling pre- and post-tests. After six months of training, significant improvement in the ability to relate phonemes to graphemes was shown by the experimental group, which even outperformed the group of students with no dyslexia.

The novelty of Nijakowska's study was that it documented how a particular instructional programme could prove successful in improving certain components of competence in a foreign language. She provided a detailed illustration of the instructional materials and gave a systematic account of the teaching and research procedures. Even though the study had only a small number of dyslexic participants, and the author was the teacher of the students, the research mainly followed the quantitative positivist paradigm, as it offered only statistical information on the students' development and little insight into the attitudes, feelings and self-perceived progress of the participants or the experiences of the teacher. Nor did the author take advantage of the possibility to present individual differences in development, because she treated her participants as a homogeneous group. As instruction to the dyslexic students was provided outside regular foreign language classes, little insight was gained into how classroom practices could be adjusted to ensure success for dyslexic language learners. Nijakowska's study exemplifies views of language learning that see development as the acquisition of linguistic knowledge (Martin, 2009). In this model of language learning, students are researched in 'laboratory contexts' and their environment is often disregarded. Development is considered a 'product' rather than a process, and is measured by isolated and decontextualised samples of language.

Studies of language use

A number of studies have been conducted on the language use of dyslexic students. Research in this field usually involves the administration of different data-collection instruments and language tests, which assess participants' knowledge and skill in producing and comprehending language. These data-collection instruments can consist either of so-called discrete-point items, in which students are expected either to choose from a set of alternatives or to provide very short answers in one isolated aspect of language competence such as grammar, or integrated tests, which aim to assess skills in language use by means of more complex tasks, such as composition writing (Alderson *et al.*, 1995). The purpose of this type of research is to describe the characteristics and level of skill in a foreign language demonstrated by dyslexic language learners (e.g. Kormos & Mikó, 2010) and to identify the strengths and weaknesses of these students (e.g. Helland, 2008; Helland & Kaasa, 2005).

Helland's (2008) and Helland and Kaasa's (2005) research projects were directed at developing an assessment tool to evaluate dyslexia-related difficulties in learning a foreign language (in Norway). Their diagnostic test consisted of a written and an oral part, contained both discrete-point and integrated tests, and measured students' oral and written language production and comprehension abilities. The test format was adjusted to the needs of dyslexic students and particular care was taken to ensure that dyslexic students enjoyed the tasks and experienced a feeling of success.

Helland (2008) found that dyslexic children with good auditory processing skills performed worse only on tests of L2 spelling, grammar and word reading when compared with students with no apparent signs of SpLDs. In contrast, dyslexic participants with poor speech perception abilities scored lower on all the components of the test, including L2 listening, speaking, vocabulary, grammar and sentence reading. She pointed out that dyslexic language learners cannot be regarded as a homogeneous group, and rightly argued that their individual cognitive profiles have to be considered carefully in instructional programmes and in assessment practices.

The innovation of Helland and Kaasa's measurement instrument was that it united expertise from the fields of special education, psychology and language research (specifically into the acquisition of a second language), and that it represented a test suited to the needs of dyslexic language learners. Importantly, the study highlighted the heterogenity and diversity of dyslexic students, which are rarely emphasised within the quantative–positivist paradigm. Nevertheless, this test development project is also an example of the biological–medical model of dyslexia, as it was based on a definition of dyslexia as a 'constitutional impairment affecting basic academic skills' (Helland & Kaasa, 2005: 54).

In the Norwegian context investigated, multilingualism meant both the acquisition of a foreign language in a classroom setting and exposure to English outside the realm of the classroom, mostly through different media channels (e.g. television and the internet). The view of language competence in this study entailed written and oral communication, which suggests that the authors regard multilingualism as a linguistic issue rather than a sociocultural phenomenon. Accordingly, the components of the test assessed spelling, vocabulary, listening comprehension, word and sentence reading, translation skills and speaking ability. The L2 test they developed was linguistic on the assumption that an initial diagnostic assessment of dyslexia that took into account the symptomatic, cognitive, biological and environmental aspects of this type of SpLD (Morton & Frith, 1995) would already be available for this group of students. Helland and Kaasa pointed out that their aim in designing the test was to assess both what students could and could not do in an L2, but they also mentioned that they wanted to gain some insight into the participants' zone of proximal development (ZPD) (Helland, 2008: 67). They argued that comparisons of students' performance in comprehending specific constructions in L2 with their ability to produce these constructions would provide information on what elements of language are present in the learner's ZPD. In Vigotsky's original conceptualisation, however, ZPD is assessed by examining what students can achieve with the help of others, including peers and teachers (Vygotsky, 1962), and not as the difference between receptive and productive knowledge.

Interview studies

In EFL contexts, several interview studies have been conducted in which teachers' and students' views and experiences with regard to the role of dyslexia in language learning were investigated. Interviews in this field, similar to the majority of studies in applied linguistics, are seen as a 'resource for investigating truths, facts, experience, beliefs, attitudes, and/ or feelings of respondents' (Talmy, 2010: 131) and serve as mere research instruments. In these studies, interview data are considered to be a truthful report of participants' feelings and experiences and are analysed 'objectively' in terms of content. Little consideration is given to the social nature of interviews, in which interviewee and interviewer collaboratively construct meaning (Silverman, 2001), or to the fact that the analysis of interview data inherently involves the interpretive stance of the researcher (Holstein & Gubrium, 2003).

Kormos and Kontra (2008) interviewed foreign language teachers and special education experts involved in a special language teaching programme for dyslexic language learners in Hungary. In-depth semi-structured interviews aimed to discover the language teachers' and special education experts' perception of the nature of the problems in learning a foreign language dyslexia causes at the classroom level. With the help of a 'thick description' of the data, the authors presented an insider's perspective of working with dyslexic language learners. The interview data revealed that teachers could recognise the manifestations of dyslexia in almost every aspect of language learning, not just in spelling and reading performance. On the basis of their findings, the authors drew up a model of teachers' perceptions of dyslexia in the process of learning a foreign language and showed how good practice in teaching foreign languages to students with SpLDs can be based on their model.

Although this study was qualitative in nature and aimed to explore how teachers in a particular instructional context perceive SpLDs, the authors' conceptualisation of dyslexia followed the biological–medical framework. The focus of their investigation was on the difficulties of learners with SpLDs at the linguistic and behavioural level in the classroom, and they highlighted the features of these learners that make them different from students with no SpLDs. Nevertheless, certain instructional and social barriers were discussed, such as the nature of the curriculum, the structure of language classes and the family environment. The model of teaching practice to be followed with students who have SpLDs, as proposed in their paper, incorporates a number of elements of sociocultural views of disability as it placed responsibility on teachers to create an instructional environment in which students with SpLDs can acquire a foreign language.

Csizér *et al.* (2010) also conducted an interview study, the aim of which was to provide an insider's account of the dynamics of the motivation to learn another language among Hungarian students with dyslexia. They based the discussion of their results on dynamic systems theory (van Geert, 1994) and argued that motivation is a dynamic characteristic of language learners that is nested in a number of systems, such as the students' immediate environment and the instructional and social setting. In this respect, the theoretical stance taken in this study shares some similarities with socio-cultural views of disabilities, which also focus on the role of social factors in creating barriers for students with SpLDs. Csizér et al. (2010) argued that the language learning motivation of students with SpLDs can fluctuate within relatively short time intervals, due to the influence of factors both external and internal to the student, and they drew up a dynamic model of language learning motivation based on their interview data with dyslexic learners. Their findings show that language learning goals, attitudes and motivation form a closely interrelated co-adaptive system, in which change in one of these motivational constructs brings about change in related constructs. They placed these motivational factors within the system of learner internal factors, which included self-perceptions and cognitive factors such as dyslexia. The learner was then situated in two interrelated external systems: milieu and instructional setting. In their research they demonstrated how influences stemming from the learners' immediate environment as well as from the instructional setting might affect learning goals, attitudes and motivation. The interviews also showed that the motivation and language learning attitudes of students with SpLDs were particularly sensitive to external influences that stem from the instructional setting. Teachers' general in-class behaviour, methods of instruction and attitudes towards dyslexia were found to have an important effect on the participants' liking of and enthusiasm for the foreign language they studied. The authors also argued that the general social context is the largest system into which all the previously mentioned subsystems need to be placed.

An innovative feature of Csizér et al.'s study was that it focused exclusively on the motivation, attitudes, experiences and feelings of students with SpLDs, without using learners with no apparent signs of learning differences as a basis for comparison. The study was also concerned with what educational barriers these learners need to face in learning a foreign language and did not highlight the difficulties that dyslexic learners as individuals have in successfully acquiring another language. Their study gave careful consideration to the instructional context and the role of students' families, and presented language learners with SpLDs as part of a dynamic system. It has to be noted, however, that the authors located dyslexia among the cognitive factors that affect language learning, and from this perspective their research also embodies elements of the biological–medical view of SpLDs. In addition, as pointed out above, neither Kormos and Kontra (2008) nor Csizér et al. (2010) considered important issues related to interviews as social practice, such as the issue of power differences between the researchers and the teachers and students interviewed, or the fact that interviewees might have more than a single voice or one coherent story to tell (Talmy, 2010).

Case studies

Case studies are the most frequently used tools in qualitative research in education (Gall *et al.*, 2003). Their aim is to provide an in-depth description of a bounded system, such as a single student, a particular group of learners, or an educational institution or programme (Creswell, 1998). Case studies provide a detailed description of a 'phenomenon in its natural context and from the perspectives of the participants involved in the phenomenon' (Gall *et al.*, 2003: 436) with the help of a variety of research tools and via multiple sources of data (Creswell, 1998).

To our knowledge, only two case studies have been conducted with dyslexic language learners in foreign language settings. In her case study of a successful dyslexic language learner, Sarkadi (2008) explored the vocabulary learning difficulties of her participant as well as her reactions to the different teaching methods that were used to help her acquire words. In another case study, Kormos *et al.* (2010) presented three instructional programmes in Hungary that have been highly successful with students with SpLDs. These case studies used a combination of research instruments, interviews, diaries and classroom observation, and a variety of data sources. They both aimed to present the language learning and instructional processes of language learners with SpLDs from an emic perspective.

The participant in Sarkadi's (2008) investigation was a Hungarian learner of English who was tutored by the author herself. Sarkadi documented the instances of her student's vocabulary learning problems in detail and thus provided an insider's view of what a dyslexic language learner experiences when studying new words in a foreign language. The study also gave an account of how multisensory techniques, explicit phonemic awareness instruction and training in language learning strategies can be used when tutoring students with SpLDs.

The novelty of Sarkadi's study was that she used various types of triangulation to gain an in-depth understanding of a single case. For data source triangulation she interviewed both the student and her parent, and for methodological triangulation she employed interviews and a teaching diary. She provided a rich description of her case by means of quotes from interviews and from her own notes made after each teaching session. Furthermore, her study also involved a prolonged observation period, as she kept records of her meetings with the student over the course of three months. In this respect, this study is an excellent example of a qualitative case study of a language learner with SpLDs. The study does, however, reflect a biological–medical view of disability, as it focuses on the nature of the difficulties the student experienced and the remedial techniques that might help the learner overcome her problems. Nevertheless, in her conclusion, Sarkadi argues that the teaching methods applied in her case study can easily be incorporated into mainstream language classrooms and consequently facilitate access to foreign language education for students with SpLDs and thus break down barriers.

The case study conducted by Kormos *et al.* (2010) examined three instructional contexts in Hungary: a publicly owned secondary school with special classes for students with SpLDs; a state-financed primary school in which students with SpLDs study foreign languages either in separate groups or in the mainstream classroom; and a privately owned secondary school which was set up for students with SpLDs. The study explicitly focused on how barriers to foreign language education are broken down and how a facilitative environment for language learning is established in these institutions. The research project used both data sources and methodological triangulation and relied on interview data gained from teachers and students as well as field notes made while observing classes. The authors succeed in presenting an insider's view of the educational practices in these three schools, with the help of quotes from the interviews and the field notes.

Despite the differences in the institutional settings and geographical locations of the schools, Kormos *et al.* found that language teaching methods and teachers' beliefs about working with students with SpLDs shared many similarities. The language teachers working with SpLDs in the investigated settings made a large number of adaptations to the syllabus and teaching materials and paid special attention to adjusting the organisation, pace and timing of language learning activities to the needs of students with SpLDs. The study also describes a large variety of techniques the participating teachers used to enhance the language learning motivation of students with SpLDs and the ways in which assessment practices were modified so that they would give a fair reflection of students' abilities in a foreign language.

From among the studies described in this chapter, this research seems to be the closest to sociocultural models of disability, in that the authors explicitly describe how socially constructed barriers to effective learning of a foreign language can be removed, at least in the Hungarian context investigated. The study also focuses on participation instead of the acquisition of linguistic knowledge, and describes how students with SpLDs are able to participate fully in foreign language education with the help of a supportive teacher and appropriate instructional methods. The study presents three special cases in Hungary, however, in which learners with SpLDs being instructed are segregated from their peers with no SpLDs. Consequently, it cannot yield insights into what happens in mainstream foreign language classes and how inclusion works in this setting.

The two case studies presented in this section can be characterised as descriptive, in that the aim is to provide a detailed a description in the hope that it will help readers understand the phenomena as they occur in context and be able to transfer the findings to their own contexts (Yin, 2003). Although they might be criticised on the ground that they did not attempt to construct a grounded theory based on their findings, these case studies might inspire further research in the field. They might also pave the way for more critical approaches to qualitative research (e.g. Pennycook, 2001) in the field that can investigate how social, political, economic and educational contexts systematically disadvantage learners with dyslexia.

Conclusion and Implications for Further Research

This chapter has reviewed the current standing of research on dyslexic language learners in European foreign language contexts. The analysis has revealed that most studies in this field have been conducted within a biological–medical framework which focuses on the source of language learning difficulties within individual learners and aims to offer treatment for the problems experienced by these students. The majority of research can also be seen to belong to the psycholinguistic paradigm, which views language learning as a cognitive process and language as a linguistic system independent of the social and cultural context. Hence quantitative investigations relying on questionnaires and linguistic analysis tend to dominate in this area of research, and consequently in most studies the researcher remains an outsider in the research context.

We do now seem to have a detailed understanding of the characteristics of 'typical' dyslexic foreign language learners in terms of their motivational, affective and cognitive profiles and the difficulties these students experience in acquiring English as a foreign language in classroom contexts. However, we have limited insight into how varied dyslexic foreign language learners are in terms of their individual characteristics and how they differ in their language learning processes. In addition, little is known about how motivational, affective and cognitive factors dynamically interact with each other and influence acquisition of a foreign language. Furthermore, no studies have yet shed light on how the instructional context influences dyslexic students' motivational and affective disposition towards the learning of a foreign language.

Research studies in this field have also been successful in describing effective language teaching programmes, but most of these instructional programmes were administered outside mainstream classes, where dyslexic language learners were taught in isolation from their peers. Furthermore, these studies were conducted in only two eastern European countries; therefore it is not clear whether their findings can be generalised to other contexts. Longitudinal research that documents the long-term effect of instructional programmes and follows students through their learning processes for an extended period of time is also scarce.

The analysis of studies in this field indicates that a paradigm shift from the biological–medical framework to a sociocultural one, and a more critical stance to research, will be necessary. Viewing SpLDs as interdependent with the social and instructional context could inspire further research that explores barriers in foreign language teaching practices, curricula and policies. The current mainly descriptive research framework would need to be complemented not only by a more exploratory approach, but also with the tools that critical applied linguistics offers, to show how students with SpLDs are disadvantaged in the context of learning a foreign language.

For this purpose, there is a need for more qualitative research methodologies, such as interviews, case studies and ethnographies, and more mixed-method studies, in which quantitative research tools are supplemented by qualitative methods of enquiry. The practices of viewing dyslexia as a cognitive individual characteristic and of conducting comparative studies of dyslexic and non-dyslexic students might need to be replaced with research that investigates dyslexic language learners as interdependent with their social, cultural and educational context. The field of second language acquisition should also show more interest in dyslexia and SpLDs and should not relegate this topic to the background, as an issue that is relevant to only a small minority of language learners.

References

Ahmad, W.I.U. (ed.) (2000) *Ethnicity, Disability and Chronic Illness*. Buckingham: Open University Press.

Alderson, J.C., Clapham, C. and Wall, D. (1995) *Language Test Construction and Evaluation*. Cambridge: Cambridge University Press.

Bandura, A. (1986) *Social Foundations of Thought and Action: A Social Cognitive Theory*. Englewood Cliffs, NJ: Prentice-Hall.

Canale, M. and Swain, M. (1980) Theoretical bases of communicative approaches to second language teaching and testing. *Applied Linguistics* 1, 1–47.

Constable, A. (2001) A psycholinguistic approach to word-finding difficulties. In J. Stackhouse and B. Wells (eds) *Children's Speech and Language Difficulties* (pp. 330–365). London: Whurr.

Creswell, J. (1998) *Qualitative Inquiry and Research Design: Choosing Among Five Traditions*. Thousand Oaks, CA: Sage.

Csizér, K., Kormos, J. and Sarkadi, Á. (2010) The dynamics of language learning attitudes and motivation: Lessons from an interview study with dyslexic language learners. *Modern Language Journal* 97, 470–487.

Department of Trade and Industry (DTI) (1995) *Disability Discrimination Act*. London: HMSO.

Dörnyei, Z. (2001) *Teaching and Researching Motivation*. London: Longman.

Dörnyei, Z. (2005) *The Psychology of the Language Learner: Individual Differences in Second Language Acquisition*. Hillsdale, NJ: Erlbaum.

Downey, D., Synder, L. and Hill, B. (2000) College students with dyslexia: Persistent linguistic deficits and foreign language learning. *Dyslexia* 6, 101–111.

Eysenck, M.W. and Calvo, M.G. (1992) Anxiety and performance: The processing efficiency theory. *Cognition and Emotion* 6, 409–434.

Gall, M.D., Gall, J.P. and Borg, W.T. (2003) *Educational Research* (7th edn). Boston, MA: Pearson Education.

Guba, E.G. and Lincoln, Y.S. (1989) *Fourth Generation Evaluation*. Newbury Park, CA: Sage.

Helland, T. (2008) Second language assessment in dyslexia: Principles and practice. In J. Kormos and E.H. Kontra (eds) *Language Learners With Special Needs: An International Perspective* (pp. 63–85). Bristol: Multilingual Matters.

Helland, T. and Kaasa, R. (2005) Dyslexia in English as a second language. *Dyslexia* 11, 41–60.

Holstein, J.A. and Gubrium, J.F. (2003) Active interviewing. In J.F. Gubrium and J.A. Holstein (eds) *Postmodern Interviewing* (pp. 67–80). Thousand Oaks, CA: Sage.

Horwitz, E.K., Horwitz, M. and Cope, J.A. (1986) Foreign language classroom anxiety. *Modern Language Journal* 70, 125–132.

Kormos, J. and Csizér, K. (2010) A comparison of the foreign language learning motivation of Hungarian dyslexic and non-dyslexic students. *International Journal of Applied Linguistics* 20, 232–250.

Kormos, J. and Kontra, H.E. (2008) Hungarian teachers' perceptions of dyslexic language learners. In J. Kormos and E.H. Kontra (eds) *Language Learners With Special needs: An International Perspective* (pp. 189–213). Bristol: Multilingual Matters.

Kormos, J. and Mikó, A. (2010) Diszlexia és az idegen-nyelvtanulás folyamata [Dyslexia and the process of second language acquisition]. In J. Kormos and K. Csizér (eds) *Rész-képességzavarok és idegen nyelvtanulás [Learning Disabilities and Foreign Language Acquisition]* (pp. 49–76). Budapest: Eötvös Kiadó.

Kormos, J., Csizér, K. and Sarkadi, Á. (2009) The language learning experiences of students with dyslexia: Lessons from an interview study. *Innovation in Language Learning and Teaching* 3, 115–130.

Kormos, J., Orosz, V. and Szatzker, O. (2010) Megfigyelések a diszlexiás nyelvtanulók idegennyelv-tanulásáról: A terepmunka tanulságai [Observations on teaching foreign languages to dyslexic students: Lessons from a field-study]. In J. Kormos and K. Csizér (eds) *Rész-képességzavarok és idegen nyelvtanulás [Learning Disabilities and Foreign Language Acquisition]* (pp. 185–211). Budapest: Eötvös Kiadó.

MacIntyre, P.D. and Gardner, R.C. (1994) The subtle effects of language anxiety on cognitive processing in the second language. *Language Learning* 44, 283–305.

Martin, D. (2009) *Language Disabilities in Cultural and Linguistic Diversity*. Bristol: Multilingual Matters.

Morton, J. and Frith, U. (1995) Causal modeling: A structural approach to developmental psychopathology. In D.J.C. Dante Cicchetti (ed.) *Developmental Psychopathology, Vol. 1: Theory and Methods* (Wiley Series on Personality Processes) (pp. 357–390). New York: Wiley.

Nijakowska, J. (2008) An experiment with direct multisensory instruction in teaching word reading and spelling to Polish dyslexic learners of English. In J. Kormos and E.H. Kontra (eds) *Language Learners With Special Needs: An International Perspective* (pp. 130–158). Bristol: Multilingual Matters.

Nijakowska, J. (2010) *Dyslexia in the Foreign Language Classroom*. Bristol: Multilingual Matters.

Pennycook, A. (2001) *Critical Applied Linguistics: A Critical Introduction*. Hillsdale, NJ: Erlbaum.

Piechurska-Kuciel, E. (2008) Input, processing and output anxiety in students with symptoms of developmental dyslexia. In J. Kormos and E.H. Kontra (eds) *Language Learners With Special Needs: An International Perspective* (pp. 86–109). Bristol: Multilingual Matters.

Sarkadi, Á. (2008) Vocabulary learning in dyslexia – The case of a Hungarian learner. In J. Kormos and E.H. Kontra (eds) *Language Learners With Special Needs: An International Perspective* (pp. 110–129). Bristol: Multilingual Matters.

Silverman, D. (2001) *Interpreting Qualitative Data: Methods for Analysing Talk, Text, and Interaction.* Thousand Oaks, CA: Sage.

Talmy, S. (2010) Qualitative interviews in applied linguistics: From research instrument to social practice. *Annual Review of Applied Linguistics* 30, 128–148.

Tobias, S. and Everson, H.T. (1997) Studying the relationship between affective and metacognitive variables. *Anxiety, Stress, and Coping* 10, 59–81.

United Nations (2006) Convention on the Rights of Persons with Disabilities. See http://www.un.org/disabilities/documents/convention/convoptprot-e.pdf (accessed 15 August 2012).

Van Geert, P. (1994) *Dynamic Systems of Development: Change Between Complexity and Chaos.* New York: Harvester Wheatsheaf.

Vinegrad, M. (1994) A revised adult dyslexia checklist. *Educare* 48, 21–23.

Vygotsky, L.S. (1962) *Thought and Language.* Cambridge, MA: MIT Press.

Yin, R. (2003) *Case Study Research: Design and Methods* (3rd edn). Thousand Oaks, CA: Sage.

5 Acquired Dyslexia in Bilingual Speakers: Implications for Models of Oral Reading

Brendan Stuart Weekes, I-Fan Su, Carol To and Anastasia Ulicheva

Introduction

A great deal of research has investigated the cognitive processes used in reading. The focus of this research has been languages that use an alphabetic script, resulting in the development of sophisticated models of oral reading in English (Coltheart *et al.*, 1993, 2001; Harm & Seidenberg, 1999, 2004; McClelland & Rumelhart, 1981; Perry *et al.*, 2007, 2010; Plaut *et al.*, 1996; Seidenberg & McClelland, 1989; Zorzi, 2010; Zorzi *et al.*, 1999) and other Indo-European languages, including German (Ziegler *et al.*, 2000). One aim of this research is to explain disorders of reading, principally dyslexia, which can result either from a failure to acquire reading skill (developmental) or loss of reading skill in adulthood (acquired). An important outcome of this work is that an understanding of the cognitive processes involved in dyslexia provides a constraint on theoretical models of oral reading. The question we ask here is whether theoretical models of oral reading can explain the patterns of acquired dyslexia observed in bilingual speakers.

To answer this question, we examine patterns of acquired dyslexia reported in bilingual speakers and show (remarkably) how they resemble acquired dyslexia reported in monolingual speakers of different languages. We then consider whether computational models of bilingual oral reading can explain these phenomena. We focus on the Bilingual Interactive Activation (BIA) model developed by Dijkstra and van Heuven (1998, 2000), which assumes an integrated system for oral reading across languages. Our conclusion is that although patterns of acquired dyslexia in bilingual speakers can be language selective in some cases, these observations do not challenge current models of reading in bilingual speakers.

First, we describe below the varieties of acquired dyslexia. Our description excludes peripheral disorders of reading (e.g. letter-by-letter reading) to focus on the theoretically relevant 'central' disorders of reading.

Acquired Dyslexia and Models of Oral Reading

Much of the progress in our current understanding of oral reading in English comes from cognitive neuropsychological studies of individuals who have disorders of reading (e.g. Valdois *et al.*, 1995; Weekes & Coltheart, 1996). For example, acquired surface dyslexia in English refers to impairment when reading aloud irregularly spelled words, particularly if words are low in frequency and have an abstract meaning, for example *indict*. This reading impairment is accompanied by a preserved ability to read regularly spelled words and non-words, for example *zint*. Surface dyslexic reading is characterised by regularisation errors in reading word components; for example, yacht is pronounced 'ya/tch/ed'. The opposite pattern of impairment is acquired phonological dyslexia, which refers to impaired reading of non-words with a preserved ability to read aloud irregularly and regularly spelled words. Acquired deep dyslexia is similar to phonological dyslexia, except the errors produced are semantic (e.g. arm → 'finger'), visual (e.g. bus → 'brush'), or morphological (e.g. run → 'running'). These patterns of acquired dyslexia are observed in Arabic, Chinese, Dutch, Finnish, French, German, Greek, Hebrew, Italian, Japanese, Mongolian, Portuguese, Slovakian, Spanish, Turkish and Welsh (Weekes, 2012). In under-studied languages such as Farsi, Devanagari, Kannada, Hindi, Korean and Russian, classification of acquired dyslexia into surface, phonological and deep is unusual (Kozintseva *et al.*, 2012). Nevertheless, case reports of bilingual speakers show that syndromes resemble patterns of acquired dyslexia reported in Indo-European languages (Byng *et al.*, 1984; Chengappa *et al.*, 2004; Karanth, 2002; Kim *et al.*, 2007; Ratnavalli *et al.*, 2000; Traugott & Dorofeeva, 2004). Although characteristics of acquired reading disorders vary across languages (and thus across scripts), such reports are of theoretical value because they demonstrate replicable patterns both within and between different language groups (Weekes, 2005).

Coltheart *et al.* (2001) proposed a 'multiple-route' model to explain oral reading and acquired disorders of reading in English. The model assumes a lexical semantic pathway available for reading aloud known words and a direct lexical pathway for reading words without contacting the meaning of that word. Coltheart *et al.* (2001) further assume a third, non-lexical grapheme-to-phoneme route, which is mandatory for reading non-words such as *zint* and is available for reading regular words but cannot support the correct reading of irregular words.

Plaut *et al.* (1996) proposed an alternative model, based on the connectionist principles of sub-symbolic processing (Seidenberg & McClelland, 1989). Critically, connectionist models eschew whole-word representations in favour of sub-word components in the onset, vowel and coda positions. Plaut *et al.* (1996) also assume two pathways but propose semantic and phonological pathways. One distinction between traditional dual-route, symbolic models and connectionist parallel distributed processing (PDP) models is that the former assume independent direct lexical and semantic pathways and connectionist models do not. In keeping with sub-symbolic representations, Plaut *et al.* (1996) also assume that non-word reading uses a process of analogy with existing sub-word representations via the non-lexical reading pathway.

Dual-route computational (DRC) and PDP models offer contrasting accounts of cases of acquired surface, phonological and deep dyslexia in English. According to Coltheart *et al.* (2001), surface dyslexia results from damage to the direct lexical or lexical semantic pathways, leading to over-reliance on the non-lexical route for reading aloud. This explains the tendency towards regularisation of irregular words using knowledge of grapheme–phoneme representations. Phonological dyslexia results from impairment to the non-lexical pathway together with preserved direct lexical and lexical semantic pathways. This explains the selective inability to read non-words. Deep dyslexia could arise from loss of lexical *and* non-lexical pathways, leading to reading by the semantic pathway (Coltheart *et al.*, 2001). According to Plaut *et al.* (1996), surface dyslexia results from impairment to the semantic pathway due to damage to representations in semantic memory as well as the bidirectional mappings between word knowledge and phonological representations. Phonological dyslexia results from severe damage to the phonological pathway, which may be abolished in deep dyslexia (Friedman, 1996).

Although the models make different predictions about the cause of impairment in acquired dyslexia, each model allows selective damage to functionally independent pathways linking orthography and phonology. Thus both models explain the variety of acquired reading disorders in English-speaking people. Both models have also been applied to explain disorders of reading in bilingual speakers – even in languages with distinctive orthographies (Béland & Mimouni, 2001; Eng & Obler, 2002; Fabbro, 1999; Raman & Weekes, 2005a, 2005b; Valdois *et al.*, 1995). However, despite the possible application of monolingual models of oral reading to explain acquired dyslexia in bilingual speakers, it is not obvious that either model can explain processes involved in bilingual oral reading. For example, it is not clear why a bilingual speaker of English and Chinese would make use of a non-lexical reading pathway, because Chinese characters cannot be read without access to a lexical representation (Weekes, 2005). For the same reason, it is not clear how purely sub-symbolic models of reading would explain the process of lexical (word-form-based) reading that is necessary to access the store of Chinese character representations needed to read aloud in Chinese.

Acquired Dyslexia in Multilingual Speakers

Studies of acquired dyslexia began over two millennia ago and progressed slowly to include bilingual speakers in the 17th century (Benton, 1964; Lordat, 1825, and Wepfer, 1690, cited in Prins & Bastiannse, 2006). In the 1960s, the Soviet neuropsychologist Alexander Luria reported a case of multilingual acquired dyslexia (Luria, 1960, cited in Kotik-Friedgut, 2006). Luria described a French journalist who had acquired dyslexia in all languages he could speak premorbidly (French, Russian, German and Polish), with greatest impairment in French. Luria noticed that the manifestation of dyslexia in each language appeared to depend on the properties of a particular script, such as regularity of the orthography-to-phonology mappings in the language. Interestingly, Luria explained the differential patterns of language impairment observed as stemming from a complex interaction of different factors, such as age of acquisition, language proficiency and language status. Luria proposed that when these factors are similar for both languages (as in early-acquired bilingualism), parallel patterns of aphasia are more likely to be observed. The question of whether the systems of oral reading in each language are dependent or independent of the type of script can be addressed only after controlling premorbid factors, as well as differences in experimental tasks (Kotik-Friedgut, 2006; Weekes et al., 2007). We return to the issue of individual differences in reading skill later in this chapter.

Wilson et al. (2012) reviewed more recent reports of acquired reading disorders in bilingual speakers (see also Obler, 1983). The review found that the error patterns of surface, phonological and deep dyslexia reported in monolingual speakers of different languages are observed in bilingual speakers of Indo-European languages, including Catalan and Spanish (García-Caballero et al., 2007), Finnish and Swedish (Laine et al., 1994), Spanish and English (Laganaro & Overton-Venet, 2001; Masterson et al., 1985), Turkish and English (Raman & Weekes, 2005a, 2005b) and Welsh and English (Beaton & Davies, 2007; Tainturier et al., 2011). This is also true for reports of bilinguals speaking two Semitic languages, Arabic and Hebrew (Friedman & Haddad, 2012; Ibrahim, 2008, 2009), as well as in comparisons across scripts that are dissimilar (Indo-European and Semitic). Béland and Mimouni (2001), for example, report the case of a speaker of both Arabic and French who presented with deep dyslexia in both languages. As in other cases of deep dyslexia, this individual produced more errors reading abstract words than concrete words, more errors on closed-class words (such as prepositions and pronouns) and more errors when reading non-words compared with words. Béland and Mimouni (2001) contrasted the DRC and the PDP connectionist models to account for patterns of reading errors observed in both languages. They noted more semantic errors in French, but more cross-linguistic errors (reading translation errors) from Arabic (i.e. a response given in French if Arabic was requested). To explain the higher rate of semantic errors in French, they assumed that phonological access to the lexicon from semantics was more impaired for French than Arabic. But, to account for translation errors from Arabic, they further assumed that access from semantics to the phonological lexicon was *unimpaired* for French. To resolve this paradox, Béland and Mimouni (2001) proposed that reading errors in their bilingual speaker resulted from a disruption to connections in an interactive activation network. To explain the differential pattern of reading errors across languages, they assumed each language shared semantic representations, so that semantically related words in French were associated with their translated equivalents in Arabic, thus leading to the production of reading translation errors. However, they also proposed independent oral reading systems for each language, with separate lesions to each system to explain dissociation in oral reading and translation errors in each language. It is important to note the key theoretical implication of their analysis, which is that multiple reading systems are necessary to explain patterns of oral reading disorder in each language. We call this the language-dependent view of reading (see also Paradis, 1994; Valdois *et al.*, 1995).

Wilson *et al.* (2012) also reported reading errors across different language types (Sino-Tibetan and Indo-European). Sino-Tibetan languages use ideographic writing systems in which the basic unit of writing (called a character) is related to a unit of meaning. One feature of these scripts compared with alphabets in Western languages is the relatively low phonological generalisability of non-alphabetic scripts; that is, scripts use a relatively arbitrary set of orthographic units to represent sounds in the language and these orthographic units do not typically give a reliable clue to the pronunciation. Other Asian languages have syllabic scripts (e.g. Japanese Kana or Indian Kannada) in which the writing system does not represent the phoneme with a single grapheme (as in alphabetic scripts) but the symbol is linked to a determined phonological unit. Wilson *et al.* found that there was little evidence to support the language-dependent view. For example, Byng *et al.* (1984) reported deep dyslexia in a speaker of English and Nepalese. Nepalese is written in the syllabic Devanagari script, which, like Japanese Kana and other south Asian syllabic scripts, requires a mapping of characters onto phonological segments (phonemes or syllables). Byng *et al.* hypothesised that the oral reading of Nepalese words written in a syllabic script would be more difficult than the oral reading of English words written in a Roman alphabet, because deep dyslexia reflects damage to the non-lexical reading pathway. They found that reading for this speaker was more difficult in Nepalese, even though it was the native, first acquired language (L1). However, further tests showed that he could understand Nepalese words written in a syllabic script as well as English words, and he could read aloud words written in the Devanagari script if he could respond in English. Byng *et al.* argued that the individual's reading difficulties in Nepalese were not due to differences in script but occurred because each script maps onto a common phonological system in different ways: directly in Nepalese and indirectly in English.

Caramelli *et al.* (1994) report a similar case of a bilingual speaker of Brazilian Portuguese and Japanese (Nisei). This man produced more oral reading errors in Japanese (ideographic) than Portuguese (alphabetic), even though he acquired both languages at an early age and was a scribe in Japanese premorbidly. Of interest was a differential pattern of reading impairment within the Japanese language for Kanji and Kana script. Japanese script uses an ideographic writing system (Kanji) adopted from Chinese characters, as well as a syllabic system (Kana). Kana is subdivided into Katakana, used for loan words, and Hiragana, used for content and function words, verb and adjective inflections, intermixed with Kanji characters. Although many case studies of monolingual Japanese speakers who can read in one script and not the other – which is called biscriptal dyslexia – have been reported (see Cremaschi & Dujovny, 1996; Iwata, 1984), the Caramelli *et al.* report was the first to show that acquired dyslexia within Japanese can transfer to irregularly spelled Portuguese words (see also Meguro *et al.*, 2003; Senaha & Parente, 2012). Such a finding is problematic for the language-dependent view, as similar patterns of acquired dyslexia and also generalisation between different scripts strongly suggest that bilingual speakers use an integrated oral reading system. We call this contrasting theoretical position the language-independent view of reading.

Consistent with the language-independent position, studies of acquired reading disorders in bilingual speakers who premorbidly read in languages with quite different scripts reveal little evidence for independent reading systems in bilingual speakers. Ratnavalli *et al.* (2000) report of bilingual speakers Kannada and English who show similar patterns of reading impairment in both languages, despite differences in features of written English and Kannada (which uses an alpha-syllabic script). Similarly, Gil and Goral (2004) report a case of a speaker of Russian and Hebrew who received treatment only in L2 (Hebrew), but after a month of therapy there had been a similar degree of improvement in his Russian as in his Hebrew. That is, despite substantial linguistic differences in the two scripts (they are written in opposite directions and differ in morphological and phonological organisation), between-language therapeutic transfer was observed and improvements were parallel for each language (see also Eviatar *et al.*, 1999). These cases suggest that language status, not type of script, produces different patterns in bilingual speakers.

Studies of bilingual speakers of Chinese and English also suggest that, although oral reading in one script (typically L1) can be more impaired than in the other following brain damage, this may be due to a selective division of labour within a common reading system. Eng and Obler (2002), for instance, observed more semantic reading errors (a characteristic of deep dyslexia) in

Chinese (L1) than English (L2). This could be interpreted as evidence for the language-dependent view, that each script is read via separate reading systems. However, an alternative explanation is that oral reading in Chinese relies more on a semantic pathway than oral reading in English. Weekes *et al.* (2007) reported bilingual speakers of Mongolian and Chinese who showed some differences in reading errors across these two scripts. The Mongolian language uses an alphabetic script (as in Indo-European and Semitic alphabets). Weekes *et al.* (2007) found better oral reading in Mongolian (L1) than Chinese (L2) and reported one person who produced semantic reading errors in Mongolian and Chinese but semantically related translation errors in Chinese only (namely, reading a Chinese character with a semantically related Mongolian syllable) and a different person who produced within-language semantic reading errors in Mongolian (e.g. 'table' read as 'stool') but did not produce such errors in Chinese. Weekes *et al.* (2007) rejected the idea of language-independent reading systems by arguing that if extraneous variables such as the age of acquisition and familiarity with words in each script are controlled, there are very few differences in the reading errors observed across each type of script, which implies the existence of a language-independent reading system.

In order to understand the patterns of acquired dyslexia in bilingual speakers, Table 5.1 presents a summary of cases reported to date that show acquired reading disorders in at least two languages. All cases are summarised in terms of the status of each language (L1 or L2), the cerebral pathology (if reported), the pattern of reading impairment and the characterisation of acquired dyslexia if stated in the case report. Note that we exclude cases of biscriptal monolingual speakers who read different scripts (e.g. Japanese), as they are not necessarily bilingual speakers.

The summary shows a mixed pattern of results with respect to the expectations of the language-dependent and the language-independent accounts of oral reading. In some cases there are no differences in quantity or quality of oral reading errors across languages, even if languages use different scripts (e.g. Arabic and Hebrew). However, in the majority of cases there is some effect of language status on performance, with a differential pattern of reading errors across languages. Two features that emerge from the summary are that: (1) the effect of language status is not necessarily in favour of the first acquired language (L1); and (2) the effect of language status does not depend on similarity between scripts. For example, there are reports of bilingual speakers of Chinese and English who produce more errors in Chinese (L1) than English (L2) (Eng, 1998; Eng & Obler, 2002) but also at least one report showing the opposite pattern (Lyman *et al.*, 1938). Similarly, reports of bilingual speakers of Arabic and Hebrew include one case with more errors in L1 (Arabic) (Ibrahim, 2008), another with more errors in L2 (Hebrew) (Ibrahim, 2009) and a third showing no difference (Friedmann & Haddad, 2012).

Table 5.1 Reported cases of dyslexia in bilingual speakers (1938–2011)

Citation	Language pairs	Neuro-pathology	Errors	Characterisation
Lyman et al. (1938)	Chinese–English	Left TBA	More reading errors in English (L2) than Chinese (L1)	None
Eng (1998)	Chinese–English	Left TBA	More reading errors in Chinese (L1) than English (L2)	Semantic errors in both languages including translation errors
Eng and Obler (2002)	Chinese–English	Left TBA	More reading errors in Chinese (L1) than English (L2)	Semantic and surface errors in both languages (stress and tonal)
Byng et al. (1984)	Devanagari–English	Left TBA	More reading errors in Devanagari (L1) than Engish (L2)	None
Kambanaros et al. (2012)	Greek–English	Left temporal CVA	More writing errors in English (L2) than Greek	Phonological dysgraphia
*Chengappa et al. (2004)	Hindi–English	None reported	More reading errors in English (L2) than in Kannada (L1)	Surface dyslexia in English
Druks et al. (2012)	Hungarian–English	Dementia (nfPPA)	More reading errors in English (L2) than Hungarian (L1)	Progressive dyslexia in both languages
Ohno et al. (2002)	Japanese–English	Left hemisphere CVA	More reading errors in Japanese than English (including translation of kana words). Writing spared	Pure alexia for Japanese Kana and Kanji
*Karanth (2002)	Kannada–English	None reported	More reading errors in English (L2) than in Kannada (L1)	Surface dysgraphia in both languages
Ratnavalli et al. (2000)	Kannada–English	Left occipital lobe	No differences between languages; writing preserved	Pure alexia in both languages (writing intact)
Ratnavalli et al. (2000)	Kannada–English	Left parietal lobe	More reading errors in Kannada (L1); writing difficulties for both languages	None
Kim et al. (2007)	Korean–English	Left hemisphere CVA	Dysgraphia in both languages transposition errors between consonants and vowels occurred in English	Graphemic buffer impairment.
Masterson et al. (1985)	Spanish–English	Left temporal CVA	More reading errors in English (L2) than Spanish (L1)	None
Laganaro and Overton-Venet (2001)	Spanish–English	Large left TBA	No differences between languages: more difficulty reading non-words compared to words	A mixture of pure and phonological alexia.
Raman and Weekes (2005a)	Turkish–English	Left temporal CVA	More reading errors in English (L2) than Turkish (L1)	Surface dyslexia in English/deep dysgraphia in Turkish

Beaton and Davies (2007)	Welsh–English	Left CVA	More reading errors in English (L2) than Welsh (L1)	Deep dyslexia in both languages
Tainturier et al. (2011)	Welsh–English	Left CVA (x7)	No difference between languages	Phonological dyslexia in both languages
García-Caballero (2007)	Galician–Spanish	Basal ganglia	Reading errors in Galician (L1) only	None
Laine et al. (1994)	Finnish–Swedish	Left anterior CVA	No differences between languages: more difficulty reading non-words compared to words	A mixture of pure and phonological alexia.
Béland and Mimouni (2001)	Arabic–French	Left temporal CVA	More reading errors in French (L2) than Arabic (L1)	Deep dyslexia in both languages
Ibrahim (2008)	Arabic–Hebrew	Left hemisphere tumour	More reading errors in Arabic (L1). Could only spell single words in Arabic	Letter-by-letter reading
Ibrahim (2009)	Arabic–Hebrew	Herpes encephalitis	More reading errors in Hebrew (L2). In spelling to dictation, Arabic better preserved than Hebrew	Letter-by-letter reading
Friedmann and Haddad (2012)	Arabic Hebrew	Left TBA	No difference between languages	Letter position dyslexia
Weekes et al. (2007)	Mongolian–Chinese	Left temporal CVA	More reading errors in Chinese (L2) than Mongolian (L1). Translation reading errors	Deep dyslexia in Mongolian and Chinese,
Meguro et al. (2003)	Portuguese–Japanese	Dementia (DAT)	More reading errors in Kanji than kana (L2) and irregularly spelled words than non-words in Portuguese (L1)	Surface dyslexia
Senaha and Parente (2012)	Portuguese–Japanese	Left traumatic brain injury	More reading errors in Kanji than kana (L2) and irregularly spelled words than non-words in Portuguese (L1)	Surface dyslexia
Caramelli et al. (1994)	Portuguese–Japanese	Left traumatic brain injury	More reading errors in Japanese (L2) than Portuguese (L1). More reading impairment for Kanji than Kana	None
Meguro et al. (2003)	Portuguese–Japanese	Dementia (Alzheimer)	Kana, Portuguese and Japanese non-words > Portuguese irregular words (L1) > Kanji characters (L2)	None
*Wydell and Butterworth (1999)	English–Japanese	None reported	More reading errors in English (L1) than Japanese (Kanji and Kana)	Developmental phonological dyslexia in English

*These are cases of developmental dyslexia where no neuropathology is reported.

CVA, cerebrovascular accident; TBA, tuberculous brain abscess; nfPPA, non-fluent variant primary progressive aphasia; DAT, dementia of the Alzheimer type.

An effect of language status on reading performance is not surprising, given that studies show one language can be more impaired than another in bilingual aphasia. It is also probable that an effect of language status is not a consequence of brain damage *per se* but reflects the premorbid proficiency with each language. Note that premorbid proficiency can be independent of the age of acquisition, as many bilingual speakers (particularly immigrants) are likely to be more proficient in the language that is more often spoken (dominant) in the home and work environment. This is particularly likely for written language, whereby *émigré* children and adults are likely to acquire literacy in the language most spoken (dominant) and perhaps not at all in the native language. If individual differences reflect premorbid reading proficiency, then this likely explains reading dissociation in bilingual speakers. This limits the inferences that can be drawn.

The BIA Model of Oral Reading in Bilingual Speakers

Unlike studies of acquired dyslexia in multilingual speakers, models of reading in bilingual speakers have a recent history. Paradis (1994) proposed the first language-dependent account of bilingual written word recognition, assuming that word forms (orthographic and phonological forms and their syntactic properties) are language specific, while conceptual features (semantic representation) are shared across language. Similarly, Kroll and colleagues assume separate lexica for L1 and L2 word forms in the Revised Hierarchical (RH) Model (Kroll & de Groot, 1997; Kroll & Stewart, 1994; though see also Kroll & Dijkstra, 2002). In the RH model, separate lexica for each language are connected via asymmetrical links according to amount of exposure (dominance or familiarity) to each language, and each lexicon of known word forms is connected to a common semantic system.

Language-independent models of bilingual written word recognition, by contrast, assume that word forms (orthographic/phonological), word meaning and conceptual features are shared in a common network for all languages. One motivation for these models comes from the observation that identical orthographic forms without any meaning relation (interlingual homographs) in L1 and L2 have an adverse effect on visual word recognition. Dijkstra and van Heuven (2002) reported an interlingual homograph effect whereby bilingual undergraduate students speaking Dutch and English took longer to accept an interlingual homograph (e.g. *room*, which means cream in Dutch) as an English word (657 ms) than to decide that a non-homograph word (e.g. *home*) was an English word (577 ms). This effect was also asymmetrical, that is, it was evident only in L2 word recognition. Further, Marian and Spivey (2003) found that among bilingual speakers of Russian and English, non-target-language items in Russian are activated during target-language processing in English if initial phonemes overlap in each language. Such findings converge on the view that representations of word forms are shared in the lexicon for bilingual speakers of languages that share a common alphabet (Dutch and English) or language family (Indo-European).

To accommodate this view, Dijkstra and colleagues developed a computational model of written word recognition called the Bilingual Interactive Activation (BIA) model (see Figure 5.1). A computational model is a mathematical model that can simulate the acquisition of culturally determined behaviour such as oral reading skill. The BIA model is an extension of the first Interactive Activation model of reading, proposed by McClelland and Rumelhart (1981), but contains levels of representation for the unique features, letters and words used in two languages that both use an alphabetic script. According to the BIA model, when a letter string is presented the

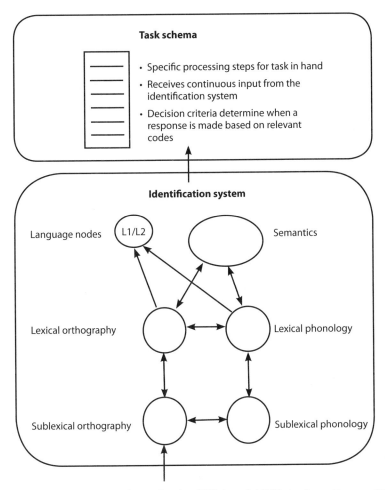

Figure 5.1 Bilingual interactive activation (BIA+) model (Dijkstra & van Heuven, 2002)

visual input activates features at each letter position, which subsequently excite letters containing features and inhibit letters for which features are absent. Activated letters then excite words in both languages, while all other words are inhibited at the word level (irrespective of language). The BIA model can explain why the statistical properties of words in one language have an effect on word recognition of similar words in the other language. This is because the model assumes an integrated lexicon for L1 and L2 orthographic word forms. The model proposed by Havelka and Rastle (2005) to explain reading in monolingual speakers who use two different scripts (biscriptal readers) makes a similar assumption about a common lexical reading pathway for oral reading in each script .

One initial criticism of the BIA model was the absence of a computational layer for phonological forms, which limits the capacity of the model to explain oral reading in bilingual speakers. Jared and Kroll (2001) reported that within-language consistency in orthography and phonology correspondences in English had an effect on oral reading of French written words in bilingual speakers. It has also been reported that oral reading performance in a target language (English) is influenced by language-specific orthographic and phonological information of the non-target language (Russian) in bilingual speakers (Kaushanskaya & Marian, 2007; Marian et al., 2008). More specifically, English non-words are read more slowly if they are 'legal' in Russian, either orthographically (letters shared in Roman and Cyrillic alphabets) or phonologically (by English letters corresponding to Russian sounds). Schwartz et al. (2007) also found negative transfer of Russian sounds on the reading development of native Russian-speaking children learning English, manifested as confusion of letter–sound correspondences.

Dijkstra and van Heuven (2002) extended their model by assuming additional (shared) phonological word forms connected to the orthographic representations and semantic features in the BIA model (see Figure 5.1). The addition of a phonological layer in the BIA+ model provided an explanation for the effects of one language on another in bilingual oral reading and the effects of one script on reading in another script in biscriptal readers. For example, Havelka and Rastle (2005) reported the effects of the Cyrillic script on the reading of the Roman script in monolingual Serbo-Croatian speakers and Rastle et al. (2009) found effects of length on reading Kanji words written in the less familiar Kana script in monolingual Japanese speakers. More critically, inclusion of a phonological layer allowed a wider range of predictions to be tested in normal and impaired bilingual speakers.

Both BIA models were designed to explain oral reading in proficient bilingual readers. However, an important constraint on the development of oral reading models in monolingual speakers comes from the capacity of a computational model to explain acquired and developmental reading problems. The assumption of integrated lexica in both BIA models predicts that disruption to oral reading will be non-selective and should produce the same pattern of impairment in both languages, particularly but not only if two scripts are similar (alphabetic, non-alphabetic, syllabic). Cross-linguistic errors in cases of acquired dyslexia in bilingual speakers (Béland & Mimouni, 2001; Byng *et al.*, 1984; Eng & Obler, 2002; Raman & Weekes, 2005a) suggest that damage to the oral reading system in bilingual speakers is non-selective and can be language independent.

The effects of language status, familiarity and dominance may be more challenging for the BIA+ model to explain. However, a computational model can accommodate these effects via changes to connection 'weights' within the model, whereby stronger weights represent more experience and greater learning; for example, early acquired and more familiar languages could be represented in the model by stronger connection weights between orthography and phonology. Note that connection weights do not need to be equivalent within languages for the connections between phonology and meaning, orthography and meaning, and orthography and phonology; this allows a bilingual speaker to be more proficient in L1 for one domain (e.g. reading) and less proficient in L1 for another (e.g. spoken word production). We argued above that the premorbid individual differences in reading proficiency of a bilingual speaker with acquired dyslexia place limitations on the theoretical interpretation of reading errors. The BIA+ model can accommodate these effects. Indeed, computational models of oral reading and acquired dyslexia incorporate these factors to extend their explanatory power to cases of acquired dyslexia in monolingual speakers (see Dilkina *et al.*, 2008).

In this approach, the premorbid abilities of individuals with acquired dyslexia are assumed to follow a normal distribution. The key feature of these models is an integrated reading system, that is, with no explicit distinction between lexical and semantic reading systems (in contrast to the DRC model). This assumption allows PDP models to explain differences in performance across cases as a consequence of normal individual differences in premorbid reading ability and preferred reading style, leading to a different division of labour across the available components of the normally developing oral reading system (see Plaut, 1997, 2002, for detailed examples). In PDP models, the components are the semantic and non-semantic (direct) pathways (Woollams *et al.*, 2007). In fact the BIA+ model assumes a semantic and a direct reading pathway. Thus, although that model can in principle explain the effects of premorbid language proficiency on reading performance in bilingual speakers, a theoretical commitment to distinguish between a lexical and a semantic reading pathway has not yet been made explicit.

Dilkina *et al.* (2008) simulated the effects of individual differences in oral reading experience by manipulating the training regime in the network and the relative 'size' of pathways mapping orthography to phonology (i.e. size of the direct pathway in the network). The term 'size' in this context refers to the number of connections between layers in the computational network and thus the capacity of the network to process increasing amounts of information. Dilkina *et al.* (2008) found the size of a pathway became larger as a consequence of experience with reading. Interestingly, individual differences explained much of the variability in overall reading impairment, as well as the variability in item-level effects in acquired reading disorders (e.g. the effects of spelling regularity in surface dyslexia). Therefore, premorbid reading experience can explain a pattern of dyslexia.

The theoretical implications of individual differences in reading experience on both skilled and impaired reading in patients with bilingual aphasia and computational models of reading in bilingual speakers are quite obvious. The effects of language status, familiarity and dominance can be simulated in the BIA+ model. Variation in reading experience with a language for a bilingual speaker can be estimated by an individual's exposure to literary texts, educational background, occupation and other demographic factors (Jared & Kroll, 2001) and modelled by adjusting the connection strengths and size of pathways within the computational model. In order to achieve this, however, BIA+ modellers need to specify whether only one pathway is necessary for reading in more than one language. The evidence from a number of language families, ranging from Indo-European to Sino-Tibetan, suggests that at least two pathways are necessary. Weekes (2005, 2012) refers to these as semantic and non-semantic reading pathways, in keeping with Coltheart *et al.* (2001); a semantic pathway is available for reading aloud known words and a non-semantic pathway is available for reading words without contacting the meaning of that word. Unlike Coltheart *et al.* (2001), however, Weekes does not assume a grapheme-to-phoneme pathway for Sino-Tibetan languages. This is because the scripts in these languages typically do not represent phonemes (as do alphabetic scripts) but represent syllables with whole characters and sub-syllabic units, such as the *mora* in Japanese Kana, with a set of orthographic units called an alpha-syllabary. It is an open question whether a non-lexical grapheme-to-phoneme pathway is actually necessary for reading alphabetic scripts and therefore it is not clear whether such a route is necessary for the BIA+ model. However, models of biscriptal oral reading do assume such a pathway and, moreover, there is evidence to suggest the operation of an independent non-lexical reading pathway with biscriptal readers (Havelka & Rastle, 2005; Rastle *et al.*, 2009).

Spelling in Bilingual Aphasia

As in oral reading, cognitive neuropsychological studies of individuals who have disorders of spelling are informative in the development of models of written word production (Weekes, 2012). For example, acquired surface dysgraphia in English refers to impairment when spelling irregularly spelled words, particularly if words are low in frequency and have an abstract meaning. This impairment is accompanied by a preserved ability to spell regularly spelled words and non-words. Surface dysgraphic spelling is characterised by regularisation errors in spelling word components; for example, yacht is written 'yot'. The opposite pattern of impairment is acquired phonological dysgraphia, which refers to impaired spelling of non-words with a preserved ability to spell irregular and regular words. Acquired deep dysgraphia is similar to phonological dysgraphia except that semantic spelling errors are produced (e.g. fruit → 'vegetable'). Another remarkable pattern is selective impairment of written spelling ability in one grammatical word class only (e.g. nouns or verbs) (Rapp *et al.*, 1997).

Acquired dysgraphia can be explained with reference to dual-route models of spelling such as that shown in Figure 5.2 (derived from Houghton & Zorzi, 2003). Such models assume that spelling relies on independent pathways. Spelling a familiar word from dictation is achieved via retrieval of a whole word from the orthographic output lexicon. The letters of a word are assembled via a graphemic output buffer (abstract representations) and a motor pattern is then activated for specific (left/right) hand movements. Dual-route models assume non-word spelling requires a non-semantic (phonological) route. Letter sequences of non-words and unfamiliar words not stored in the orthographic lexicon and are assembled via knowledge of sound–spelling correspondences and by learned rules that are used to assemble graphemes for writing in a sequential order (Miceli & Capasso, 2006).

Acquired dysgraphia has been reported mostly in Indo-European languages but is also observed in Chinese speakers (Law *et al.*, 2005; Leung *et al.*, 2012). Reports of acquired dysgraphia in bilingual speakers are rare but notable. Raman and Weekes (2005b) reported a patient who had deep dysgraphia in Turkish (L1) and English (L2) characterised by impairments to non-word spelling, written picture naming in both languages and poor spelling of homophones in English. There was also an effect of grammatical class on spelling in Turkish, with nouns spelled better than verbs (see also Weekes & Raman, 2008). Raman and Weekes argued that spelling deficits in bilingual individuals with deep dysgraphia result from partial damage to a semantic spelling pathway (left-hand side of the model in Figure 5.2) and complete damage to the non-lexical phonological route (right-hand side of the model in Figure 5.2). Raman and Weekes (2005b) also proposed a language-independent account of bilingual dysgraphia; that is, each pathway was used to spell both languages and spelling was not constrained by the specific linguistic properties of a language. This account of bilingual dysgraphia assumes that spelling of words and non-words in both languages relies on a common system and, if damaged, similar patterns of dysgraphia will be observed in each language.

Kambanaros and Weekes (2013) tested this language-independent hypothesis with a bilingual speaker of Greek and English who showed a similar

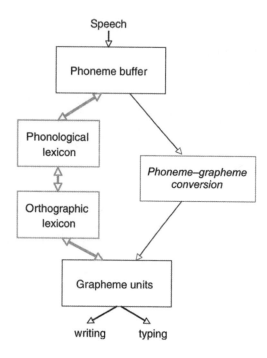

Figure 5.2 Model of spelling (derived from Houghton & Zorzi, 2003)

pattern of acquired phonological dysgraphia when spelling non-words in the two languages. As in many other cases of phonological dysgraphia, there was an effect of grammatical class on spelling. Surprisingly, however, English nouns were spelled better than English verbs and the reverse pattern was seen in Greek (Greek verbs spelled better than Greek nouns). Differential effects of grammatical class on word spelling in each language suggest that lexical spelling of verbs and of nouns in phonological dysgraphia *is* constrained by the linguistic properties of each language, contrary to the language-independent hypothesis. Specifically, verb spelling is less vulnerable than noun spelling in Greek, whereas verbs are more vulnerable than nouns in English. Furthermore, Kambanaros *et al.* (2012) compared spoken and written naming performance in this same individual and found there was more difficulty retrieving written object names than action names in Greek but there were no differences between actions and objects in English written naming. In addition, written word naming was better than spoken word naming in both languages.

How can retrieval of spoken words be more impaired than retrieval of written words in a bilingual person with dysgraphia and why are there different effects of grammatical class on spelling in bilingual dysgraphia? All cognitive models of lexical retrieval assume that spoken and written word production share conceptual representations but have different output mechanisms. To retrieve a picture name, the speaker must identify an action or object (e.g. a picture of scissors) and recognise the concept to be named. This is considered a pre-semantic stage of processing. Next, a name is retrieved after the concept is distinguished visually and semantically. This is the lexical–semantic stage. It is at this stage that morphosyntactic information first becomes available. In English and Greek, for example, 'scissors' is a single noun, but in Greek it also comes with neuter gender. Finally, the word form of a concept is retrieved. For spoken word production, the corresponding representation of the sound of the word that is stored in the phonological output lexicon is retrieved and instructions are given to the sensorimotor system to coordinate and produce speech sounds for oral word production. For written naming, a corresponding orthographic form is retrieved from the orthographic output lexicon, which activates the graphemic patterns for written output, including allograph selection, retrieval of graphic motor patterns and motoric execution (Weekes, 1994).

The orthographic autonomy hypothesis (OAH) assumes that the orthographic representations for written picture naming are directly retrieved without phonological mediation (Rapp et al., 1997). According to the OAH, grammatical class effects in written word production could be observed without grammatical class effects on spoken word production because the phonological output lexicon and orthographic output lexicon are independent systems in the language network (see Figure 5.2). This explains why spoken word retrieval can be more impaired than written word retrieval in a bilingual person with dysgraphia and why different effects of grammatical class can be observed on spelling in bilingual dysgraphia.

No model of dysgraphia can account for differences in patterns of preserved and impaired spelling across languages in a bilingual speaker. Such patterns of dysgraphia are also problematic for the language-independent hypothesis of spelling in bilingual dysgraphia (Raman & Weekes, 2005b). According to the dual-route model in Figure 5.2, one locus of grammatical class effects in bilingual dysgraphia is the semantic pathway, since this is where morphological knowledge is represented. Kambanaros and Weekes (2013) argued that morphological differences between English and Greek are represented in this pathway because Greek is a stem-based language with a complex morphology, making information about grammatical category and morpho-syntactic word features more prominent. Therefore, grammatical knowledge can affect the orthographic retrieval of Greek nouns because spelling via language-specific processes is required. This account of the grammatical class effect on writing in Greek is compatible with one assumption of the OAH, namely that retrieval of orthography depends on grammatical function, and is also compatible with dissociations in written spelling in morphologically rich languages such as Spanish (Iribarren *et al.*, 2001; Wilson *et al.*, 2007) and Italian (Angelelli *et al.*, 2004) as well as in Sino-Tibetan languages (Lam *et al.*, 2012).

The selective effects of grammatical class on spelling for Greek–English and Turkish–English cases of acquired dysgraphia can also be accounted for according to the model in Figure 5.2. Dissociations between action and object naming are observed in bilingual speakers typically in both languages spoken (Hernández *et al.*, 2007, 2008). Such findings can be taken as evidence for the claim that words are organised in the language system according to semantic and grammatical categories. A small group of studies has reported an effect of word class on written picture naming of actions and objects in individuals with aphasia. In these cases, the writing performance of patients was spared relative to spoken word production (Rapp & Caramazza, 2002). However, a selective deficit for actions can be restricted to writing in some patients and restricted to speech in others (Caramazza & Hillis, 1991), or a selective deficit for objects can be seen in speech only (Hillis & Caramazza, 1995). Most intriguingly, the same patient may have difficulty with verbs in spoken but not written word production and with nouns in written but not spoken word production (Rapp & Caramaza, 2002). Such results suggest there are in the brain modality-specific (spoken or written) components for both input and output available for writing verbs and nouns (Hillis & Caramazza, 1995). Hernández *et al.* (2008) described the spoken and written output of a bilingual speaker with word-finding difficulties due to degenerative neuropathology. Before the onset of the illness, the patient was highly proficient in Spanish and Catalan. When he was presented with the same set of action and object pictures, selected to elicit noun and verb production during spoken and written output, he performed better on object than action words in both modalities and both languages, albeit worse in Catalan (L2). The dissociation between action and object naming in written and spoken word output supports the hypothesis that the grammatical categories of verbs and nouns are shared for cognitive and neural mechanisms across languages in bilingual speakers (Miozzo *et al.*, 2010).

Closing Remarks

We have known for over 2000 years (since Valerius Maximus) that damage to the brain can result in reading disorder and for over 300 years that reading impairment can be more severe in one language than another in a bilingual speaker (Lordat, 1825, cited in Critchley, 1964). It is now becoming clear why the cognitive processes in oral reading become selectively impaired both within and between languages. Our review shows that data from acquired dyslexia in bilingual speakers can be accommodated in a computational framework such as the BIA+ model if the weights on nodes in an integrated reading system are assumed to be strong for frequently encountered words. Although we contend that greater association strength in the weights of a computational model should reflect language dominance, an alternative hypothesis is that age of acquisition of a language is also a constraint. It is possible, in principle, for a second acquired language to dominate the connection weights between orthography and phonology within an integrated lexicon if exposure to L2 is greater over the life span, as, for example, might be the case with *émigré* readers. The BIA+ model does not distinguish between the age of acquisition and frequency of exposure to written word forms. We cannot reject the age-of-acquisition hypothesis. However, cases in Table 5.1 show that reading impairment can be greater in the first acquired language. It is important to note that most reports typically do not state the age of acquisition of reading skill in a language. Tests of the age-of-acquisition hypothesis should carefully control for correlations between the age of acquisition and the frequency of exposure to a language over the life span.

One implication for modelling acquired dyslexia in bilingual speakers is that language-selective effects need not reflect different lexica or the operation of independent reading systems between or within languages. Surface dyslexia can be lack of reading experience in one language, as in developmental dyslexia (Ziegler & Goswami, 2005).

Current computational models of oral reading in English are language specific. These models share several assumptions with the BIA+ model; for instance, learning is assumed to be via a strengthening of the connections between information nodes that represent unique features of orthographic and phonological units in a language. Plaut (1997) showed that differences in script could be instantiated in a PDP model by adjusting connection weights to reflect the relative consistency in mappings between orthography and phonology in a language. The BIA+ model is a computational framework in which all written words are processed on the basis of similarity between word form representations in an integrated lexicon (as in monolingual models). The critical distinction of the BIA+ model is that oral reading in a bilingual person activates a common set of orthographic units, regardless of differences in script. Our review of the extant data in acquired dyslexia supports this assumption, even when the languages of a bilingual speaker use different orthographies. Models of bilingual reading can therefore accommodate acquired dyslexia in bilingual speakers.

Current computational models of spelling in English are also language specific. There is no computational model of bilingual spelling available to interpret acquired dysgraphia in bilingual speakers. However, the evidence suggests that even though phonological spelling is language independent (Kambanaros & Weekes, 2012; Raman & Weekes, 2005b; Tainturier *et al.*, 2011), the spelling of verbs and nouns in bilingual dysgraphia can reveal differences in the morphological and grammatical features of each of the languages used by a bilingual speaker and that these are most likely

represented in a semantic pathway. To explain why the grammatical properties of each language constrain spelling in bilingual phonological dysgraphia,
future computational models of both normal and impaired spelling must
consider how the properties of a language constrain spelling in the semantic
pathway.

References

Angelelli, P., Judica, A., Spinelli, D., Zoccolotti, P. and Luzatti, C. (2004) Characteristics
    of writing disorders in Italian dyslexic children. *Cognitive and Behavioral Neurology* 17,
    18–31.
Beaton, A. and Davies, W. (2007) Semantic errors in deep dyslexia: Does orthographic
    depth matter? *Cognitive Neuropsychology* 24 (3), 312–323.
Béland, R. and Mimouni, Z. (2001) Deep dyslexia in the two languages of an Arabic/
    French bilingual patient. *Cognition* 82, 77–126.
Benton, A.L. (1964) Contributions to aphasia before Broca. *Cortex* 1, 314–327.
Byng, S., Coltheart, M., Masterson, J., Riddoch, J. and Prior, M. (1984) Bilingual biscriptal
    deep dyslexia. *Quarterly Journal of Experimental Psychology A: Human Experimental
    Psychology* 36A (3), 417–433.
Caramazza, A. and Hillis, A. (1991) Lexical organization of nouns and verbs in the brain.
    Nature 349, 788–790.
Caramelli, P., Parente, M., Hosogi, M.L., Bois, M. and Lecours, A.R. (1994) Unexpected
    reading dissociation in a Brazilian Nisei with crossed aphasia. *Behavioural Neurology*
    7, 156–164.
Chengappa, S., Bhat, S. and Padakannaya, P. (2004) Reading and writing skills in
    multilingual/multiliterate aphasics: Two case studies. *Reading and Writing: An Inter-
    disciplinary Journal* 17 (1–2), 121–135.
Coltheart, M., Curtis, B., Atkins, P. and Haller, M. (1993) Models of reading aloud:
    Dual-route and parallel-processing-distributed approaches. *Psychological Review* 100,
    589–608.
Coltheart, M., Rastle, K., Perry, C., Langdon, R. and Ziegler, J. (2001) DRC: A dual route
    cascaded model of visual word recognition and reading aloud. *Psychological Review* 108
    (1), 204–256.
Cremaschi, F. and Dujovny, E. (1996) Japanese language and brain localization. *Neurologi-
    cal Research* 18 (3), 212–216.
Critchley, M. (1964) *Developmental Dyslexia*. London: Heinemann.
Dijkstra, A. and van Heuven, W.J.B. (1998) The BIA model and bilingual word recognition.
    In J. Grainger and A. Jacobs (eds) *Localist Connectionist Approaches to Human Cognition*
    (pp. 189–225). Hillsdale, NJ: Erlbaum.
Dijkstra, T. and van Heuven, W.J.B. (2002) The architecture of the bilingual word recogni-
    tion system: From identification to decision. *Bilingualism: Language and Cognition* 5,
    175–197.
Dilkina, K., McClelland, J. L. and Plaut, D.C. (2008) A single-system account of semantic
    and lexical deficits in five semantic dementia patients. *Cognitive Neuropsychology* 25,
    136–164.
Druks, J., Aydelott, J., Genethliou, M., Jacobs, H. and Weekes, B.S. (2012) Progressive
    dyslexia: Evidence from Hungarian and English. *Behavioural Neurology* 25 (3), 185–191.
Eng, N. (1998) Reading disruptions in a Chinese-English reader following TBI. Paper
    presented at the Advanced Studies Institute, Neuro and Cognitive Science of the
    Chinese Language, University of Hong Kong.

Eng, N. and Obler, L.K. (2002) Acquired dyslexia in a biscript reader following traumatic brain injury: A second case. *Topics in Language Disorders* 22 (5), 5–19.

Eviatar, Z., Leikin, M. and Ibrahim, R. (1999) Phonological processing of second language phonemes: A selective deficit in a bilingual aphasic. *Language Learning* 49 (1), 121–141.

Fabbro, F. (1999) *The Neurolinguistics of Bilingualism: An Introduction.* Hove: Psychology Press.

Friedman, R.B. (1996) Recovery from deep alexia to phonological alexia: Points on a continuum. *Brain and Language* 52, 114–128.

Friedmann, N. and Haddad, M. (2012) Letter position dyslexia in Arabic: From form to position. *Behavioural Neurology* 25 (3), 193–203.

García-Caballero, A., García-Lado, I., González-Hermida, J., Area, R., Recimil, M.J., Juncos Rabadán, O., Lamas, S., Ozaita, G. and Jorge, F.J. (2007) Paradoxical recovery in a bilingual patient with aphasia after right capsuloputaminal infarction. *Journal of Neurology, Neurosurgery, and Psychiatry* 78, 89–91.

Gil, M. and Goral, M. (2004) Nonparallel recovery in bilingual aphasia: Effects of language choice, language proficiency, and treatment. *International Journal of Bilingualism* 8 (2), 191–219.

Harm, M.W. and Seidenberg, M.S. (1999) Phonology, reading acquisition, and dyslexia: Insights from connectionist models. *Psychological Review* 106, 491–528.

Harm, M.W. and Seidenberg, M.S. (2004) Computing the meanings of words in reading: Cooperative division of labour between visual and phonological processes. *Psychological Review* 111, 662–720.

Havelka, J. and Rastle, K. (2005) The assemble of phonology from print is serial and subject to strategic control: Evidence from Serbian. *Journal of Experimental Psychology: Learning, Memory and Cognition* 31(1), 148–158.

Hernández, M., Costa, A., Sebastián-Gallés, N., Juncadella, M. and Reñe, R. (2007) The organization of nouns and verbs in bilingual speakers: A case of bilingual grammatical category-specific deficit. *Journal of Neurolinguistics* 20, 285–305.

Hernández, M., Caño, A., Costa, A., Sebastián-Gallés, N., Juncadella, M. and Gascón–Bayarri, J. (2008) Grammatical category-specific deficits in bilingual aphasia. *Brain and Language* 107, 68–80.

Hillis, A.E. and Caramazza, A. (1995) Representation of grammatical categories of words in the brain. *Journal of Cognitive Neuroscience* 7, 457–458.

Houghton, G. and Zorzi, M. (2003) Normal and impaired spelling in a connectionist dual-route architecture. *Cognitive Neuropsychology* 20, 115–162.

Ibrahim, R. (2008) Performance in L1 and L2 observed in Arabic–Hebrew bilingual aphasic following brain tumor: A case constitutes double dissociation. *Psychology Research and Behaviour Management* 1, 11–19.

Ibrahim, R. (2009) Selective deficit of second language: A case study of a brain-damaged Arabic–Hebrew bilingual patient. *Behavioral and Brain Functions* 12, 5–17.

Iribarren, C.I., Jarema, G. and Lecours, R.A. (2001) Two different dysgraphic syndromes in a regular orthography, Spanish. *Brain and Language* 77, 166–175.

Iwata, M. (1984) Kanji versus kana: Neuropsychological correlates of the Japanese writing system. *Trends in Neuroscience* 7, 290–293.

Jared, D. and Kroll, J.F. (2001) Do bilinguals activate phonological representations in one or both of their languages when naming words? *Journal of Memory and Language* 44, 2–31.

Kambanaros, M. and Weekes, B.S. (2013) Phonological dysgraphia in bilingual aphasia: Evidence from a case study of Greek and English. *Aphasiology* 27 (1), 59–79.

Kambanaros, M., Messinis, L. and Anyfantis, E. (2012) Bilingual lexical access in the naming and writing of action and object words. *Behavioural Neurology* 25, 215–222.

Karanth, P. (2002) The search for deep dyslexia in a syllabic script. *Journal of Neurolinguistics* 15 (2), 143–155.

Kaushanskaya, M. and Marian, V. (2007) Bilingual language processing and interference in bilinguals: Evidence from eye tracking and picture naming. *Language Learning* 57 (1), 119–163.

Kim, H., Na, D.L. and Park, E.S. (2007) Intransigent vowel–consonant position in Korean dysgraphia: Evidence of spatial-constructive representation. *Behavioural Neurology* 18, 91–97.

Kotik-Friedgut, B. (2006) Development of the Lurian approach: A cultural neurolinguistic perspective. *Neuropsychology Review* 16 (1), 43–52.

Kozintseva, E., Skwortsow, A., Ulicheva, A. and Vlasova, A. (2012) Cognitive structure of writing disorders in Russian: What would Luria say? *Behavioural Neurology* 25, 1–10.

Kroll, J.F. and de Groot, A.M.B. (1997) Lexical and conceptual memory in bilinguals: Mapping form to meaning in two languages. In A.M.B. de Groot and J.F. Kroll (eds) *Tutorials in Bilingualism: Psycholinguistic Perspectives* (pp. 169–199). Hillsdale, NJ: Erlbaum.

Kroll, J.F. and Dijkstra, A. (2002) The bilingual lexicon. In R. Kaplan (ed.) *Handbook of Applied Linguistics* (pp. 301–321). Oxford: Oxford University Press.

Kroll, J.F. and Stewart, E. (1994) Category interference in translation and picture naming: Evidence for asymmetric connections between bilingual memory representations. *Journal of Memory and Language* 33, 149–174.

Laganaro, M. and Overton-Venet, M. (2001) Acquired alexia in multilingual aphasia and computer-assisted treatment in both languages: Issues of generalisation and transfer. *Folia Phoniatrica et Logoaedica* 53, 135–144.

Laine, M., Neimi, P., Neimi, J. and Koivuselkä-Sallinen, P. (1990) Semantic errors in deep dyslexia. *Brain and Language* 38, 207–214.

Laine, M., Niemi, J., Koivuselkä-Sallinen, P., Ahlsén, E. and Hyönä, J. (1994) A neuro-linguistic analysis of morphological deficits in a Finnish–Swedish bilingual aphasic. *Clinical Linguistics and Phonetics* 8, 177–200.

Lam, K., Weekes, B.S., Kong, A.P.H. and Abutalebi, J. (2012) Impaired word retrieval in aphasia: A trilingual case study. *Procedia*, 204–205.

Law, S.-P., Yeung, O., Wong, W. and Chiu, K.M.-Y. (2005) Processing of semantic radicals in writing Chinese characters: Data from a Chinese dysgraphic patient. *Cognitive Neuropsychology* 22 (7), 885–903.

Leung, M.-T., Law, S.-P., Fung, R., Lui, H.-M. and Weekes, B. S. (2012) A model of writing Chinese characters: Data from acquired dysgraphia and writing development. In E. Grigorenko, E. Mambrino and D. Preiss (eds) *Writing: A Mosaic of New Perspectives* (pp. 357–370). Hove: Psychology Press.

Lyman, R.S., Kwan, S.T. and Chao, W.H. (1938) Left occipito-parietal brain tumour with observations on alexia and agraphia in Chinese and English. *Chinese Medical Journal* 54, 491–515.

Marian, V. and Spivey, M. (2003) Bilingual and monolingual processing of competing lexical items. *Applied Psycholinguistics* 24, 173–193.

Marian, V., Blumenfeld, H. and Boukrina, O. (2008) Sensitivity to phonological similarity within and across languages. *Journal of Psycholinguistic Research* 37(3), 141–170.

Masterson, J., Coltheart, M. and Meara, P. (1985) Surface dyslexia in a language without irregularly-spelled words. In K. Patterson, J.C. Marshall and M. Coltheart (eds) *Surface Dyslexia: Cognitive and Neurological Studies of Phonological Reading*. Hillsdale, NJ: Erlbaum.

McClelland, J.L. and Rumelhart, D.E. (1981) An interactive-activation model of context effects in better perception, Part 1: An account of basic findings. *Psychological Review* 88, 375–405.

Meguro, M., Senaha, M.L.H., Caramelli, P., Ishizaki, J., Chubacci, R.Y.S., Ambo, H., Nitrini, R. and Yamadori, A. (2003) Language deterioration in four Japanese–Portuguese bilingual patients with Alzheimer's disease: A trans-cultural study of Japanese elderly immigrants in Brazil. *Psychogeriatrics* 3 (2), 63–68.

Miceli, G. and Capasso, R. (2006) Spelling and dysgraphia. *Cognitive Neuropsychology* 23, 110–134.

Miozzo, M., Costa, A., Hernandez, M. and Rapp, B. (2010) Lexical processing in the bilingual brain: Evidence from grammatical/morphological deficits. *Aphasiology* 24, 262–287.

Obler, L.K. (1983) Dyslexia in bilinguals. In R.N. Malatesha and H.A. Whitaker (eds) *Dyslexia: A Global Issue* (pp. 477–496). The Hague: Martineau and Nijhoff.

Ohno, T., Takeda, K., Kato, S. and Hirai, S. (2002) Pure alexia in a Japanese-English bilingual: Dissociation between the two languages. *Journal of Neurology* 249, 105–107.

Paradis, M. (1994) Neurolinguistic aspects of implicit and explicit memory: Implications for bilingualism and second language acquisition. In N.C. Ellis (ed.) *Implicit and Explicit Learning of Languages* (pp. 393–419). London: Academic Press.

Perry, C., Ziegler, J.C. and Zorzi, M. (2007) Nested incremental modeling in the development of computational theories: The CDP+ model of reading aloud. *Psychological Review* 114 (2), 273—315.

Perry, C., Ziegler, J.C. and Zorzi, M. (2010) Beyond single syllables: Large-scale modeling of reading aloud with the Connectionist Dual Process (CDP++) model. *Cognitive Psychology* 61 (2), 106–151.

Plaut, D.C. (1997) Structure and function in the lexical system: Insights from distributed models of word reading and lexical decision. *Language and Cognitive Processes* 12 (5/6), 765–805.

Plaut, D.C. (2002) Graded modality-specific specialization in semantics: A computational account of optic aphasia. *Cognitive Neuropsychology* 19 (7), 603–639.

Plaut, D.C., McClelland, J.D., Seidenberg, M.S. and Patterson, K. (1996) Understanding normal and impaired word reading: Computational principles in quasi-regular domains. *Psychological Review* 103, 56–115.

Prins, R. and Bastiannse, R. (2006) The early history of aphasia. *Aphasiology* 20 (8), 762–791.

Raman, I. and Weekes, B.S. (2005a) Acquired dyslexia in a Turkish–English speaker. *Annals of Dyslexia* 55 (1), 71–96.

Raman, I. and Weekes, B.S. (2005b) Deep dysgraphia in Turkish. *Behavioural Neurology* 16, 1–11.

Rapp, B. and Caramazza, A., (2002) Selective difficulties with spoken nouns and written verbs: A single case study. *Journal of Neurolinguistics* 15, 373–402.

Rapp, B., Benzing, L. and Caramazza, A. (1997) The autonomy of lexical orthography. *Cognitive Neuropsychology* 14, 71–104.

Rastle, K., Havelka, J., Wydell, T., Coltheart, M. and Besner, D. (2009) The cross-script length effect: Further evidence challenging PDP models of reading aloud. *Journal of Experimental Psychology: Learning, Memory and Cognition* 35 (1), 238–246.

Ratnavalli, E., Geetha Murthyb, G., Nagarajaa, D., Veerendrakumara, M., Jayaramb, M. and Jayakumarc, P.N. (2000) Alexia in Indian bilinguals. *Journal of Neurolinguistics* 13, 37–46.

Schwartz, M., Geva, E., Leikin, M. and Share, D.L. (2007) Learning to read in English as L3: The cross-linguistic transfer of phonological processing skills. *Written Language and Literacy* 10 (1), 25–52.

Seidenberg M.S. and McClelland, J.L. (1989) A distributed, developmental model of word recognition and naming. *Psychological Review* 96, 523–568.

Senaha, M.L.H. and Parente, M.A.M.P. (2012) Acquired dyslexia in three writing systems: Study of a Portuguese–Japanese bilingual aphasic patient. *Behavioural Neurology* 25 (3), 255–272.

Tainturier, M.J., Roberts, J., Schiemenz, S. and Leek, E.C. (2011) Do reading processes differ in transparent vs. opaque orthographies? A study of acquired dyslexia in Welsh/English bilinguals. *Cognitive Neuropsychology* 28 (8), 546–563.

Traugott, N.N. and Dorofeeva, S.A. (2004) To the problem of impairment of reading in patients with aphasia. *Journal of Evolutionary Biochemistry and Physiology* 40 (5), 471–480.

Valdois, S., Cabonnel, S., David, D., Rousset, S. and Pellat, J. (1995) Confrontation of PDP models and dual route models through the analysis of a case of deep dysphasia. *Cognitive Neuropsychology* 12, 681–724.

Weekes, B.S. (1994) A cognitive-neuropsychological analysis of allograph errors from a patient with acquired dysgraphia. *Aphasiology* 8 (5), 409–425.

Weekes, B.S. (2005) Acquired disorders of reading and writing: Cross-script comparisons. *Behavioural Neurology* 16 (2–3), 51–57.

Weekes, B.S. (2012) Acquired dyslexia and dysgraphia across scripts. *Behavioural Neurology* 25, 159–163.

Weekes, B.S. and Coltheart, M. (1996) Surface dyslexia and surface dysgraphia: Treatment studies and their theoretical implications. *Cognitive Neuropsychology* 13, 277–315.

Weekes, B.S. and Raman, I. (2008) Bilingual deep dysphasia. *Cognitive Neuropsychology* 25, 411–436.

Weekes, B.S., Su, I-F., Yin, W-G. and Zhang, X-H. (2007) Oral reading in bilingual aphasia: Evidence from Mongolian and Chinese. *Bilingualism: Language and Cognition* 10 (2), 201–210.

Wilson, M.A., Martinez-Cuitino, A.M., Defior, S. and Weekes, B.S. (2007) Dissociable effects of grammatical class in acquired dysgraphia: Evidence from Spanish. *Brain and Language* 103, 30–31.

Wilson, M.A., Kahlaoui, K. and Weekes, B.S. (2012) Acquired dyslexia and dysgraphia in bilinguals across alphabetical and non-alphabetical scripts. In M. Gitterman, M. Goral and L. Obler (eds) *Aspects of Multilingual Aphasia* (pp. 187–204). Bristol: Multilingual Matters.

Woollams, A.M., Lambon Ralph, M.A., Plaut, D.C. and Patterson, K. (2007) SD-squared: On the association between semantic dementia and surface dyslexia. *Psychological Review* 114 (2), 316–339.

Wydell, T.N. and Butterworth, B.L. (1999) A case study of an English–Japanese bilingual with monolingual dyslexia. *Cognition* 70, 273–305.

Ziegler, J. and Goswami, U. (2005) Reading acquisition, developmental dyslexia, and skilled reading across languages: A psycholinguistic grain size theory. *Psychological Bulletin* 131 (1), 3–29.

Ziegler, J.C., Perry, C. and Coltheart, M. (2000) The DRC model of visual word recognition and reading aloud: An extension to German. *European Journal of Cognitive Psychology* 12, 413–430.

Zorzi, M. (2010) The connectionist dual process (CDP) approach to modelling reading aloud. *European Journal of Cognitive Psychology* 22 (5), 836–860.

Zorzi, M., Houghton, G. and Butterworth, B. (1999) Two routes or one in reading aloud? A connectionist dual-process model. *Journal of Experimental Psychology: Human Perception and Performance* 24 (4), 1131–1161.

6 Implementation of National Policy on Dyslexia in the Teaching of English as a Foreign Language

Maria Rontou

Introduction

Establishing a commitment to 'Education for All', the Salamanca statement produced by the United Nations Educational, Scientific and Cultural Organization (UNESCO) declared that children with special educational needs 'must have access to regular schools' in order to combat discriminatory attitudes, build an inclusive society and achieve education for all (UNESCO, 1994). The practice of accommodation and modification of the regular curriculum contributes to fairer access to education for all students. In the context of dyslexia, accommodations are a set of arrangements to ensure students with dyslexia can demonstrate their strengths and abilities (Crombie, 2002, cited in Reid, 2009). This chapter reports a study of two schools' accommodations in relation to oral examinations for students with a diagnosis of dyslexia.

National guidelines in Greece produced by the Ministry of National Education and Religious Affairs (MNERA) require teachers to use the same exam paper and to examine *verbally*, not in writing, students with dyslexia, with the same questions as their peers (MNERA, 2009; Ministry of Education, Lifelong Learning and Religious Affairs, 2010). These arrangements aim to accommodate the additional needs of students with dyslexia and to support them to perform as well as they can in exams. The curriculum for English as a foreign language (EFL) in Greek secondary schools presents an additional challenge for learners with dyslexia, as it involves a different orthography from the Greek. The oral accommodation in EFL exams therefore has heightened salience for students with dyslexia.

In this chapter I discuss a theoretical and methodological approach to investigate organisational relationships in an emerging system of educational provision for students with dyslexia. I describe an ethnographic case study of managing EFL teaching and learning with four students with dyslexia in two Greek state secondary schools. Specific issues are discussed concerning the arrangements for oral examination of students with dyslexia and the relationship between schools and diagnostic centres.

Much research on learning, particularly in special educational needs (SEN), focuses on individual learning. Here our focus of study is joint learning activity within a school in the process of implementation of accommodations of oral exams for specific learners. The conceptual framework is sociocultural activity theory. An analysis of systemic contradictions identifies levels of breakdown in the implementation of national policy for students with dyslexia in EFL provision, in Greece. In the following section we offer a historical and cultural background to the Greek educational legislative context for SEN. We then present key concepts of sociocultural activity theory and apply them in an analysis of systemic dilemmas that occur in two schools in their implementation of oral exams as stipulated in the national policy of accommodation for EFL learners with dyslexia.

The Greek Educational System

This section presents the historical context of Greek educational policy on SEN and dyslexia, specifically the administration of Greek education and policy making by the MNERA (Figure 6.1). This discussion provides a context for the analysis of the data presented in this chapter.

Pigiaki (1999) argues that because Greek education has adopted a highly centralised and hierarchical system, every important decision is decided within the MNERA, which is the apex of the system, and teachers are expected simply to implement those decisions (see Figure 6.1). The Greek Ministry of National Education and Religious Affairs changed its name to the Ministry of Education, Religion and Lifelong Learning after the change of the government at the end of 2009.

The Directorates of Primary and Secondary Education in 54 prefectures are involved in the administration of education at regional level (Ifanti, 1995; MNERA, 1983; see Figure 6.1). A Director of Education is responsible for the coordination of education in each prefecture and the supervision of head-teachers (Ifanti, 1995). At a local level, head-teachers are responsible for the implementation of policies disseminated to schools, and schools are run by the teaching staff and representatives from the local authorities, parents and students' communities (Constantopoulou, 2002; MNERA, 1985). Quality control of the educational process in schools is the responsibility of advisers in primary and secondary education. In secondary education each school adviser is responsible for a group of teachers who teach in the same discipline, and provide in-service training and pedagogic support for them (Ifanti, 1995).

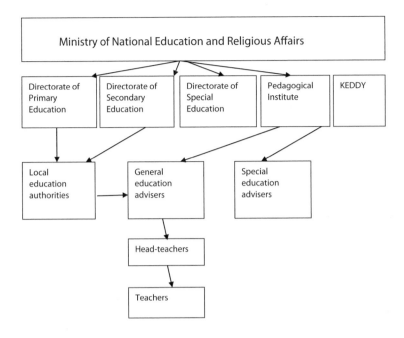

Figure 6.1 The Greek education system (adapted from Lappas, 1997)

Accommodations

Regular school programmes have accommodations to allow students with SEN to participate to their fullest extent. Accommodations can include curriculum changes and supplementary equipment; in relation to this study, one accommodation is to allow students with difficulties in reading and writing to answer exam questions orally instead of in writing, and another is to place easily distracted students in smaller, quieter classrooms. Greek education policy specifies sets of arrangements to ensure students with dyslexia can demonstrate their strengths and abilities. The following discussion reviews research and policies for SEN, in particular dyslexia, in Greece, focusing on accommodations for oral exams for students with dyslexia.

Special Education: Policy and Provision in Greece

Legislation in Greece in 2000 required centres for the diagnosis, assessment and support of students with SEN (KDAY) to be established at the seats of the prefectures (city/town education authorities). The centres function as independent state services that are directly responsible to the

Minister of Education (MNERA, 2000). The purpose of these centres is to assess students with SEN, support, inform and raise awareness in teachers, parents and wider society, and collaborate with the special needs advisers. Their purpose also includes creating adapted individualised programmes of support in collaboration with teachers and special educational staff (MNERA, 2000, 2008). KDAY became KEDDY under more recent law, but the centres still provide support for various SEN diagnoses, including guidelines for teachers (MNERA, 2008, 2009), although, as noted below, this is not always provided.

Students with a diagnosis of dyslexia are given the option to be examined orally in school tests during the school year and in end-of-year exams. The oral tests during the year are conducted by the class teacher while the final exams are conducted by two teachers in the same curriculum discipline. These students also have the option to write the answers to questions (Ministry of Education, Lifelong Learning and Religious Affairs, 2010).

Research indicates constraints on the efficiency of this provision. KEDDY centres responsible for assessment and support of students with SEN are still too few to meet the needs of all students. They are concentrated in the big urban centres (MNERA, 1994) and as a result they have long waiting lists (Haralabakis, 2005; Markou, 1993; MNERA, 1991; Nikolopoulou, 1986). Furthermore, there is a lack of specialist staff and especially of educationists (Constantopoulou, 2002; Haralabakis, 2005; MNERA, 1994). Despite the law on SEN, the diagnostic assessments of SEN given by these centres do not often lead to teaching guidance, any reference to educational programmes or any reference to collaboration between the medico-pedagogical centres and teachers (MNERA, 2000; Constantopoulou, 2002).

Studies exploring collaboration across professional groups in Greece have found a largely profession-discrete approach to SEN and dyslexia. Assessment of students with SEN, including dyslexia, is carried out by specialist professionals, such as school/educational psychologists. The relationship between schools, teachers and psychologists is complex. One Greek study (Gavrilidou et al., 1994) has shown that Greek elementary school teachers and undergraduate teacher trainees consider school psychologists to be useful in helping them solve classroom problems, while trainees rate psychologists as more useful for conduct problems than for learning problems. Evidence suggests that there are no specialist teachers or SEN school advisers at secondary school level to support teachers (Constantopoulou, 2002) and teachers report a lack of contact and collaboration with other professionals (Arapogianni, 2003).

Research studies in Greece find that teachers are aware of accommodations policy requirement allowing students with dyslexia to take exams orally (Arapogianni, 2003). However, Constantopoulou (2002) found in a study of mainstream secondary schools that differentiation of the curriculum for students with dyslexia was absent, possibly because there were no specialist teachers or SEN school advisers to offer support. Nevertheless, a range of differentiation and accommodation practices for students with dyslexia are reported to be used in schools, including oral examination, extra time in class and in exams, sensitive marking and differentiated homework (Arapogianni, 2003; Lappas, 1997; Nijakowska, 2000).

This review of contemporary special education and policies in Greece identifies a historical perspective and the implications for policy implementation. The concept of and provision for SEN is relatively recent in Greece, and it appears there may be inconsistent implementation of education policy that provides for accommodations for students with dyslexia.

Theoretical Frame: Sociocultural Activity Theory

A fundamental concept of Vygotskian ideas of learning is the joint activity, rather than individual action, of those involved in the learning task. It is most frequently represented in the 'basic mediational triangle' (Cole, 1996). An important development of Vygotskian ideas of learning is the application of these concepts to collaborative learning in groups and organisations to achieve 'formative interventions in the workplace' (Engeström, 2007: 363). Engeström expanded the basic mediational triangle by including macro-level relationships to represent other knowledges that act upon the participants, their focus of change and learning, and their learning activity. Engeström (2001) describes how current understanding of activity theory (AT) has evolved through three generations of research. The first-generation model of collective learning relations concerns the notion of 'mediation' (Vygotsky, 1987) (Figure 6.2), where the learning relationship concerns how two or more individuals (subjects) negotiate and achieve their shared goal (object) through the resources they bring (mediating artefacts/tools) (Engeström, 2001). First-generation activity theory in this study analyses instances of one-to-one learning that resolves shared dilemmas between EFL teachers and pupils in EFL exam accommodation arrangements.

Activity (learning) carried out by the subject includes an object, tools and the outcome. The subject is the group whose actions are analysed in the

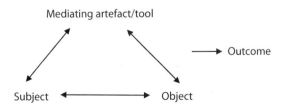

Figure 6.2 Basic mediational model proposed in first-generation activity theory

activity system (Daniels, 2004). The object of an activity is explored by the subject group according to their goal of activity (Bedny & Harris, 2005), so that the object is the shared problem and focus of learning for the subject group (Martin, 2008), and the outcome, or goal, is the joint resolution of the shared problem.

The subject–object interaction is mediated by tools, which are the resources available to the subject (Bedny & Harris, 2005). Tools are categorised by their mediational function in resolving the problem: what, how, why, and where to. 'What' tools are the products that mediate problem resolution; 'how' tools are the processes and procedures that mediate within or between objects; 'why' tools are the rationales and circumstances that mediate change; and 'where to' tools are plans and policies that mediate changes for future trajectories (Cole, 1996; Engeström, 1999a).

Second-generation activity theory: Organisational learning

The first generation focused on individuals' learning. For the second generation, developed from Leont'ev's writings (Leont'ev, 1978, 1981), Engeström (2001) expanded the basic representation of an activity system of individual actors mediating with tools, to enable examination of activity systems at an organisational level (Daniels, 2004). This expansion of the Vygotskian triangle represents the macro-level of organisational elements in an activity system. Three specific additional elements that are concerned with the same object are 'community', 'rules' and 'division of labour', and these need to be considered in problem resolution (Leadbetter, 2004; Daniels, 2004).

Second-generation activity theory analyses the complex interactions that generate and resolve problems at an organisational level in the workplace. The expanded activity system includes macro-relations between the subject and organisation, represented at the baseline (community, rules, and division of labour) in Figure 6.3. Community is the associated people

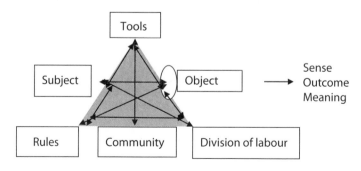

Figure 6.3 Mediation model from second-generation activity theory

and sociocultural discourses involved with the problem (object); rules are the principles, written and unwritten, regulating the actions of participants; and division of labour is the distribution of the workload (Daniels, 2004). Problems are mediated by tools across the whole organisational activity system.

In this expanded activity system, learning is collective rather than individual (Engeström, 2001). The organisation's activity system is the unit of analysis for learning (Martin, 2008). In Figure 6.3, the double-headed arrows show that all elements of the activity system are related to each other. A change in one of the elements leads to a change in the activity system as a whole (Virkkunen & Kuutti, 2000). The goal in an activity system is to generate 'creative effort' in order to resolve problems (Davydov, 1999).

Contradictions

Contradictions are problems, tensions and dilemmas encountered by participants in the course of trying to achieve an effective product or service. They arise from the processes within and between the elements of the activity system and become the object of collaborative learning, to be resolved to improve organisational performance. It is widely accepted that internal contradictions are the driving force of change and development in activity systems (Il'enkov, 1977, 1982, cited Engeström, 2001). In this study, second-generation AT analyses contradictions that emerge in the implementation of national policy on accommodations for dyslexia needs in EFL provision in two secondary schools in Greece.

Further, Engeström expands second-generation AT by drawing on Bakhtin's (1981, 1986) ideas of dialogicality and multi-voicedness (Engeström, 2001; Daniels, 2004). Multi-voicedness is used in this study to identify and analyse multiple points of view on the same issue, from the participants (EFL teachers, students, parents, head-teachers) and policy documents from the Ministry of Education. The object of learning is the accommodation for oral examination in EFL exams.

Third-generation activity theory: Learning across multiple activity systems

Third-generation AT, proposed by Engeström (2001), develops conceptual tools to analyse relationships in networks of interacting activity systems. He expands the framework of second-generation AT to include two or more interacting activity systems (see Figure 6.4). Engeström directs his analysis towards how the 'object' is created from the contradictions and tensions across networks of interacting activity systems (Daniels, 2004). Joint activity on the object/objects is needed to achieve an outcome. Evidence is drawn from dialogue and multiple perspectives. In this study,

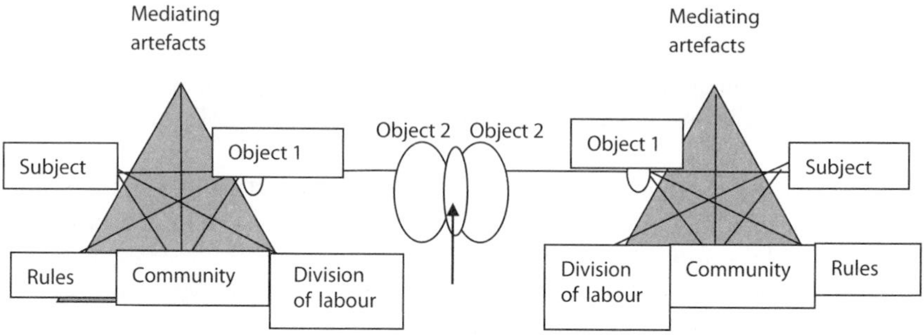

Figure 6.4 Two interacting systems as a minimal model for third-generation activity theory

third-generation AT is used to analyse the absence of joint working across the activity systems of schools and a state diagnostic centre in a Greek education authority.

In Figure 6.4, object 1 is the initial state of the focus of learning in each activity system, but each object 1 has not yet been reflected on collectively across the activity systems. In this study, school 1 represents one activity system, and the subject group comprises the EFL teachers and the students with dyslexia whom they teach, and their object 1 might be construed as resolving a problem around arranging oral exams for learners with dyslexia. The second activity system is the specialist diagnostic centre and the subject group comprises psychologists, who focus on achieving their own object 1, for example resolving the problem of workload in completing diagnostic assessments of students with dyslexia. Object 2 is constructed by expanded activity of the subject groups of the two interacting activity systems. For example, two object 2s in this study might be to assess students with dyslexia at school and to communicate diagnostic information and teaching guidance about students to schools.

Further expanded joint working by the two subject groups realises object 3, a shared object, jointly constructed by the two interacting activity systems (Engeström, 2001). Object 3 in this context might be to co-construct differentiated teaching and assessment for students with dyslexia. No evidence was available in this study of interacting activity systems to support an analysis of third-generation AT learning.

The Case Study

The two research questions concerned the schools' activity systems in implementing the national policy:

(1) What contradictions arise in the secondary schools in making formal arrangements to implement the oral exam policy?

(2) How do EFL teachers implement the national policy for secondary students with diagnoses of dyslexia?

Case study design is often used where AT forms the theoretical framework (e.g. Engeström, 1999a, 1999b, 2001) and draws on multiple sources of data collection (Denscombe, 2003). The data were collected through ethnographic methods of iterative interviews, observations, audio-recorded class lessons and field notes.

Data collection involved two schools in a city in Greece: school 1 (S1), an upper secondary school; and school 2 (S2), a lower secondary school. Participants in S1 were a 17-year-old boy, George (not his real name), his mother and father (M1 and F1), his EFL teacher (T1)and the head-teacher of the school (HT1). George was in the second year of senior high school. He had been diagnosed with dyslexia at the age of 14. He had EFL lessons up to B class at a language school but then he stopped because he did not have time and he did not like it. T1 had 19 years of teaching experience, six years of which were in the state sector. HT1 had taken up the role of head-teacher that year in the school, where he had previously been a teacher of Greek.

The data collection in S2 involved three boys aged 13, Stathis, Petros and Thodoris (not their real names), their parents, their EFL teacher (T2) and the head-teacher (HT2). The students attended the low-ability EFL class in the school. In addition, they attended out-of-school EFL classes. Stathis attended EFL lessons at a language school for C class. Petros attended private lessons for A class at home. Thodoris attended EFL lessons at a language school for B class. T2 had 19 years of teaching experience, eight years of which were in the state sector. HT2, who was previously a teacher of Greek, had been in the role of head-teacher for two or three years. The subjects in the activity systems of both schools are the EFL teachers, the head-teachers, four students with diagnoses of dyslexia, George, Petros, Stathis and Thodoris, and their parents.

Accommodations for oral exams in EFL exams

The Ministry of Education's guidelines (MNERA, 2009; Ministry of Education, Lifelong Learning and Religious Affairs, 2010) require teachers to orally examine students with dyslexia on the same exam questions as their peers. These arrangements aim to accommodate the additional needs of students with dyslexia and to support them to perform as well as they can in exams. The EFL curriculum in Greek secondary schools presents an additional challenge for learners with dyslexia, as it involves a different orthography. For these reasons, the oral exam accommodation in EFL exams would have additional salience for students with dyslexia. Where there is no school policy, how do teachers interpret and implement the national policy for students with diagnoses of dyslexia?

In this section, the unit of analysis is the activity system in each school. In response to the two research questions, there are three analyses for the contradictions that arise implementing the EFL oral exam for students with dyslexia. Selected data present the perspectives of teachers, students and parents regarding arrangements for accommodations for oral EFL exams in both schools. Analysis specifically concerns identification of the systemic contradictions evidenced in tensions and dilemmas articulated in interviews with the participants concerning arrangements for the oral exams.

School 1 (S1)

Data in S1 came from T1, HT1, a student named George, and his father on the issue of timetable arrangements for the oral examination of students with dyslexia. T1's aim was to orally examine George in EFL during the school year according to the Ministry of Education's policy. In her data extract below, from an interview with the author (MR), she reports that she gave George the opportunity to be examined orally on his chosen EFL exam questions, by taking him aside and telling him that since she had not finished marking his written paper he still had the opportunity to improve his grade with his oral exam. George did not to turn up and she felt that it was George's responsibility to do so, and not hers to chase him. She agreed that arranging the time for the oral exam with George was difficult (although it is not said, one explanation is that the oral exams are not planned in the school timetable) and she accepted MR's suggestion that George may be shy or embarrassed about discussing these arrangements in front of other pupils, although it was and would be just the two of them:

T1: Quite simply there wasn't a grade because I was waiting.
MR: To come and tell you.
T1: To come and have a re-examination as well.
MR: Why didn't he come?
T1: But he didn't come and I can't be after him when we have told him that he has this option.
MR: And how can the time be found?
T1: Yes, it is difficult but I had taken him aside and I had talked to him in private.
MR: Maybe he is shy.
T1: Eh? Okay, but it would be me and him it wouldn't be, it wouldn't be in front of….

It would seem that the oral exam is not only not timetabled by the school, nor pre-planned between the teacher and George, but that it is arranged soto voce with George to avoid his embarrassment. Yet George is entitled to this arrangement to support his academic achievement and it is a requirement for the school and teachers.

George's parents also wanted the oral exams for their son. They complained that when they had visited the teachers in school after George's first term, they did not seem to be aware of George's needs, or of the necessary arrangements to comply with the policy, so they had not arranged to orally examine George and they did not do so.

> **M1:** Not only did they not know that there was a problem, that is, ... when we went George was completing his first four months [a term] and they hadn't even gone to the trouble of telling him 'come to tell us orally'.

In the same interview, George's father (F1) and mother (M1) described a similar scenario that had occurred in the previous and current years with the history teacher, who had not accommodated George's needs with an oral exam. The parents indicated that lack of accommodation with oral exams across academic curriculum subjects was not uncommon in George's experience in the school.

> **F1:** Last year, while he was writing his history exam, he says 'can I say it orally?' because George will make a mistake. 'It doesn't matter George', she says. Why doesn't it matter?
> **M1:** 'It doesn't matter, George', she says, 'instead of 18 you get 15'. 'Why did I get 15?' 'Because there is no clear meaning' ... 'I can tell you orally', 'eh now? [How can we do it?]
> **MR:** When did this happen?
> **M1:** Now, now, this has happened now as well.
> **MR:** With teachers of Greek?
> **M1:** I can't remember if it happened with a teacher of Greek. It has happened with a theoretical subject in which you could have an oral exam, that is, in economics and in business management. It has happened sometime.

In interviews with George it is clear he also wanted the oral exams:

> **G:** I have one simple problem – it would be better for me to be examined orally.

George thought it was unfair that teachers treated him as a typical student who could write. While they might know about his dyslexia, he felt they do not know how to accommodate his difficulties either in marking his written work or by giving him an oral exam. He felt he should be given the opportunity to be examined orally in exams during the year:

> **MR:** You would like some information to be available to teachers so that...

George: Okay, teachers know about it but they don't all know how they should…

MR: correct [your work]…

George: No. Okay, to correct as well. Okay. They think of me as a student who writes. Normally they should take me out and then give me the exam orally.

In a later interview with MR, at George's house, he said he was determined to go and give some answers orally to the EFL teacher (T1):

George: I will go and give her [T1] the answers orally, whenever I can.

Although George was aware that this was not always a successful strategy, as on a previous occasion had not been able to find the EFL teacher in time:

George: She gave us the exam paper today when we had the lesson. We had to write Ancient Greek. Afterwards I didn't get to her.…

Indeed, George was planning to suggest doing the oral exam in place of his physical education (PE) lesson:

George: I will probably go during a PE lesson because I can't miss another subject.

Later, in conversation with his father, George showed that he was not pleased with the option he had suggested of doing the oral exam in place of his PE lesson, but he felt he had no option:

F1: Will you miss the PE lesson?

George: What can I do? I have to [laughing].

In a field note of her interview with HT1, MR noted his awareness of the difficulty in finding time for the oral examination of students with dyslexia, although the requirement was better met in the end-of-year exams:

I asked how students with dyslexia are examined in exams during the year. He said they can write and then give the answers orally and I asked 'Does it take place during the break or do they arrange another time for it?' He said it isn't very easy but it takes place during the final exams.

MR's field notes give the impression that the oral exam accommodations for students with dyslexia seem to be left to personal arrangements; and while HT1 reinforces the perception of the difficulty of arranging the

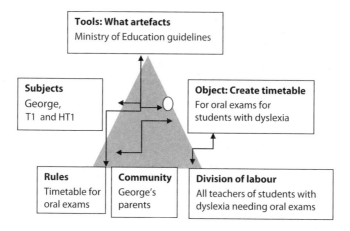

Figure 6.5 Contradictions in the activity system for oral examinations in school 1

accommodations, he confirms that the oral exam accommodations do take place at least once a year.

The data from key players (subject), George, the EFL teacher and the head-teacher evidence a contradiction in the accommodation of oral exams in the school timetable (rules). George's parents (community) support this contradiction (see Figure 6.5). Intervention for the contradiction would mediate a new process for oral exam accommodation in the school, which would be a 'how' tool, to effect changes in the timetable. It is important too that the contradiction is not shared by all teachers within the school's activity system (division of labour). An intervention may also need to work on developing raised awareness about accommodation across the staff before working to resolve the main contradiction.

If an intervention phase were added to this study, it would involve collective problem solving by S1's subject group to resolve the contradiction of arranging oral exams. The subject group might collectively create a new object that identified the need to create a school timetable that included oral exam arrangements. Further joint activity could achieve an inclusive exam timetable (see Figure 6.6).

George and T1 tried to resolve the problem at the level of individual action (Figure 6.7) but their individual action did not (indeed, could not) resolve the organisational contradiction. Through their personal agency they mediated a short-term solution based on conducting the oral exam during a PE lesson. Figure 6.7 represents the basic mediation model between George and T1 representing their attempt to resolve the problem of arranging a time for

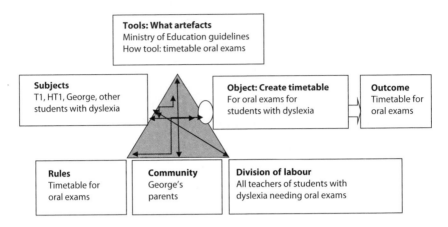

Figure 6.6 New object for T1 and George

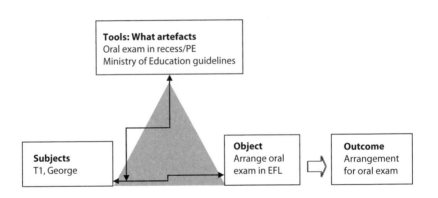

Figure 6.7 The EFL teacher (T1) and George arrange the oral exam in EFL: The basic (first-generation) mediation model

the EFL oral exam. Yet the short-term solution did not resolve the problem because further organisational problems prevented their arrangement for the oral exam. Recognising that personal initiative and agency in themselves are not sufficient to resolve organisational contradictions is an important finding. Individual agency must be harnessed to shared goals and outcomes at an organisational level to resolve the dilemmas in a sustainable way.

School 2

The systemic contradiction concerning additional arrangements for verbal examination of the written exams, including EFL, also appears in the S2 data. Evidence from T2, three of her students and a parent (Petros's mother, M3) reflects this dilemma. The data are presented so that the position of T2 is established first, and the perspectives of the students with dyslexia and one of their parents follow, as these were in response to T2's position.

T2's policy for students with dyslexia who need to answer orally some exercises in a written EFL exam was to keep them in during the breaks to do so, or at the end of the day:

> **MR:** If you see that they need to give some answers verbally do you keep them in during the break?
>
> **T2:** Of course. If they want to be examined verbally I keep them in.

The three students with dyslexia objected to this arrangement (which was used for other subjects as well as), partly because of the potentially negative impact on their assessment (see below). Stathis, for example, disagreed with the oral exam taking place during break or at the end of the day because there was not enough time for either, as he had other lessons to go to:

> **MR:** So you can simply write what you can and you can stay at the end of the day?
>
> **Stathis:** You know what, there is rarely any time during the break or at the end of the day, you know, because at 2.30 I have other lessons so I can hardly make it....

Similarly, Petros complained that the oral exam was inadequate when it was conducted at the end of the day. When T2 arranged the last oral exam for the end of the day, Petros was tired and he had forgotten the answers by then:

> **Petros:** In this exam she gave us the teaching hour to write it, and when it was over I still had an exercise left to do. She said 'come and do it orally'.
>
> **MR:** Did you do it?
>
> **Petros:** I did it but it was after the last teaching hour and I had forgotten them a bit and I didn't....
>
> **MR:** ... At the end of the day that is?
>
> **Petros:** Yes, yes, because we wrote the exam at the fourth I think or fifth hour and after the seventh hour when we had religious education and the other teacher had tired us; she tells me and the other two boys 'come and give me your answers orally' and we didn't do well at all.

Thodoris, like Stathis and Petros, did not like the oral exam to take place at the end of the day. He did not like being on his own and he felt that he was delaying the teacher as she conducted the oral exam for them, and it made him anxious. He preferred to have the oral exam when he was with his class:

> **Thodoris:** ... I want ... to see more children so I can say 'great, I have time', that is, not to delay the teacher, that is, I want the teacher to call me at the end of the day ... and tell me 'come and give me the answers orally'... I see Miss only and I think 'what am I doing here, only [me] with the teacher?' When there are more children I feel better.
> **MR:** Okay, if there are two more is that better? If there are more children from other classes?
> **Thodoris:** I like it with more children.
> **MR:** When you are with your whole class.
> **Thodoris:** Yes, I like this much more.

Stathis complained that a two-week delay between the written and oral exams in French meant he would have forgotten the answers for the oral exam:

> **Stathis:** It is a little difficult because, for example, we wrote French on Wednesday two weeks ago.
> **MR:** Yes.
> **Stathis:** And I haven't taken the oral exam yet.
> **MR:** Perhaps at the end of the school day?
> **Stathis:** But I have forgotten them [the answers] and there is no way I can write [remember] them again.

Stathis also suggested an alternative arrangement for the oral exam, whereby it took place while the other students completed their written exam, on condition that the other students were not allowed to talk or be disruptive so that the students with dyslexia could think:

> **Stathis:** The only option is to do it during the lesson while the others are writing but the others should not be allowed to ask questions, to talk or to make a noise at that time so that the others can think.

Thodoris also did not mind taking the oral exam while his classmates wrote the exam:

> **Thodoris:** I personally don't mind if the whole class is writing the exam and Miss takes me to her desk so that I give her the [spoken] answers.

The students' antagonism to the oral exam taking place in the break was echoed by the one of the parents. Petros's mother also disapproved of the EFL oral exam being conducted during the break because she felt the students needed their break and there was noise outside the classroom:

MR: … she [the EFL teacher] does it during the break as far as I understood.

M3: Because in Greek they [the other students] don't leave [the classroom] in all subjects and again at the break they want to run, [they want] to go to play or they hear the noise going on outside during the break so it works somewhat negatively.

She also thought that the oral examination should not take place at the end of the day either, because the students were tired by then:

MR: Could he stay at the end of the day or would he be tired?

M3: After seven hours … you are [tired]. They have religious education twice a week at the seventh teaching hour and when they write at that time and they take longer to finish; you can see all the children are [tired].

Figure 6.8 summarises the activity system at S2 around the contradiction arising from the arrangements for the EFL oral exams. The subject group, T2, Stathis, Petros and Thodoris, create the contradiction, while the students and a parent from S2's community agree in their concerns about the tensions generated by the arrangements to meet the requirement to allow for an oral exam in EFL. The lack of a suitable timetable or some other

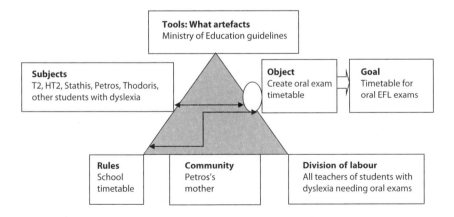

Figure 6.8 New object for participants at school 2

'how' tool (rules) gives rise to a dilemma. The oral exam, as envisaged in the national policy, should allow students with dyslexia to perform optimally, yet the existing oral exam arrangements provided by staff (during break, at the end of the day or in class while classmates write the exam) do not allow for optimal performance according to the students and parents.

Both schools' activity systems generated contradictions around the arrangements for oral exams arrived at by similarly constituted subject groups: T1 and a student in S1, and T2 and students in S2. Furthermore, in both schools parents contributed to voicing the contradiction and echoing the student perspective.

In Figure 6.8 we also present an analysis of the expanded learning needed in S2's activity system to resolve the contradictions to meet the MNERA's requirement to implement oral exams across curriculum areas for students with a diagnosis of dyslexia. The absence of collective learning around the dilemmas, as in S1, drove the EFL teacher and students with dyslexia in S2 to use their personal agency to mediate *ad hoc* arrangements for the oral EFL exam. Students and parents agreed that these arrangements were not fit for purpose, principally because of insufficient time during recess, and fatigue and anxiety at the end of the school day.

Summary

(1) What contradictions arise in the secondary schools in making formal arrangements to implement the oral exam policy?
(2) How do EFL teachers implement the national policy for secondary students with diagnoses of dyslexia?

Analysis of the evidence using two generations of AT shows similar findings across the two schools. The failure in both schools to organise systemically for the MNERA's requirement for accommodation through oral exams drove key participants, namely the EFL teachers and students with dyslexia, to individual action to mediate solutions to the problem by arranging oral exams in EFL in break and after school.

The result of individual action through a 'basic mediation triangle' was short-term expediency, which did not effect systemic change and which was not always successful, due to systemic or personal constraints. Specific constraints articulated by the students with dyslexia illustrated that oral exams in break and after school actually exacerbated the students' dyslexia and learning difficulties and diminished their assessment performance.

Figures 6.6 and 6.8 presented analyses of an expanded activity system for both schools, which identified systemic dilemmas and possible solutions, namely the development of a new school timetable. A new inclusive timetable would create a rule to organise teachers' and students' resources, such as time in the school day and classroom space, in order to meet the legal requirement for oral subject exams for students with a diagnosis of dyslexia that would be fit for purpose.

Analyses of local historical/cultural practices may identify further contradictions in the schools' activity systems. The introduction of the requirement to orally examine this specific group of learners is relatively recent, and schools may experience some inertia in organising new systemic arrangements. In addition, the effect of initiatives from the MNERA in terms of training or guidance to schools and staff, or penalties for non-compliance, was not yet evident in this study. The study sought to capture a range of perspectives, particularly from the young students and their parents, and has given a rich and powerful insight into their learning needs.

The introduction to the chapter noted that two important features of AT have not been included in this study. Third-generation AT, which incorporates joint organisational learning, was not included because there is limited evidence of joint learning across interacting activity systems between schools and the specialist education provision centres. The second aspect of AT not included in this study is intervention to change and develop further the joint collective learning in the activity systems in the schools and specialist provision. This aspect of study is more feasible with a research team than in research by a single doctoral researcher. Nevertheless, during this study there were indications of awareness-raising among the individual participants – teachers, head-teachers, parents and students. Future studies that choose this context to apply AT could consider how intervention might be accomplished, for example by developing tools to encourage second-generation activity joint working within schools with appropriate 'how' tools to implement policies to support students with dyslexia and other SEN in inclusive education contexts.

References

Arapogianni, A. (2003) Investigating the approaches that teachers in Greece use to meet the needs of children with dyslexia in secondary schools. Unpublished MA thesis, University of Birmingham.

Bakhtin, M.M. (1981) *The Dialogic Imagination: Four Essays by M.M. Bakhtin*. Austin, TX: University of Texas Press.

Bakhtin, M.M. (1986) *Speech Genres and Other Late Essays*. Austin, TX: University of Texas Press.

Bedny, G.Z. and Harris, S.R. (2005) The systemic-structural theory of activity: Applications to the study of human work. *Mind, Culture and Activity* 12 (2), 128–147.

Cole, M. (1996) *Cultural Psychology: A Once and Future Discipline*. Cambridge, MA: Harvard University Press.

Constantopoulou, X. (2002) *Educational Policy and Practice for Dyslexic Pupils: The Greek Case*. Athens: Educational Issues Publishers.

Crombie, M. (2002) Dyslexia: A new dawn. Unpublished PhD thesis, University of Strathclyde.

Daniels, H. (2004) Activity theory, discourse and Bernstein. *Educational Review* 56 (2), 121–132.

Davydov, V.V. (1999) The content and unsolved problems of activity theory. In Y. Engestrom, R. Miettinen and R.L. Punamaki (eds) *Perspectives on Activity Theory* (pp. 39–51). Cambridge: Cambridge University Press.

Denscombe, M. (2003) *The Good Research Guide for Small-Scale Social Research Projects* (2nd edn). Maidenhead: Open University Press.

Diniz, F.A. and Reed, S. (2001) Inclusion – The issues. In L. Peer and G. Reid (eds) *Dyslexia – Successful Inclusion in the Secondary School* (pp. 26–34). London: David Fulton Publishers.

Engeström, Y. (1999a) Activity theory and individual and social transformation. In Y. Engeström, R. Miettinen and R.L. Punamaki (eds) *Perspectives on Activity Theory* (pp. 19–38). Cambridge: Cambridge University Press.

Engeström, Y. (1999b) Innovative learning in work teams: Analysing cycles of knowledge creation in practice. In Y. Engeström, R. Miettinen and R.L. Punamaki (eds) *Perspectives on Activity Theory* (pp. 377–404). Cambridge: Cambridge University Press.

Engeström, Y. (2001) Expansive learning at work: Toward an activity theoretical reconceptualization. *Journal of Education and Work* 14 (1), 133–156.

Engeström, Y. (2007) Putting Vygotsky to work: The change laboratory as application of double stimulation. In H. Daniels, M. Cole and J. Wertsch (eds) *The Cambridge Companion to Vygotsky* (pp. 363–382). Cambridge: Cambridge University Press.

Ganschow, L., Schneider, E. and Evers, T. (2000) Difficulties of English as a foreign language (EFL) for students with language-learning disabilities (dyslexia). In L. Peer and G. Reid (eds) *Multilingualism, Literacy and Dyslexia* (pp. 182–191). London: David Fulton Publishers.

Gavrilidou, M., De Mesquita, P.B. and Mason, E.J. (1994) Greek teachers' perceptions of school psychologists in solving classroom problems. *Journal of School Psychology* 32 (3), 293–304.

Haralabakis, M. (2005) Three years in the lists of shame: In the margin children with learning difficulties until they are assessed. *Ta Nea*, 17 February, p. 15.

Ifanti, A. (1995) Policy making, politics and administration in education in Greece. *Educational Management and Administration* 23 (4), 271–278.

Il'enkov, E.V. (1977) *Dialectical Logic: Essays in its History and Theory*. Moscow: Progress.

Il'enkov, E.V. (1982) *The Dialectics of the Abstract and the Concrete in Marx's 'Capital'*. Moscow: Progress.

Lappas, N. (1997) Specific learning difficulties in Scotland and Greece: Perceptions and provision. Unpublished PhD thesis, University of Stirling.

Leadbetter, J. (2004) The role of mediating artefacts in the work of educational psychologists during consultative conversations in schools. *Educational Review* 56 (2), 133–145.

Leont'ev, A.N. (1978) *Activity, Consciousness, and Personality*. Englewood Cliffs, NJ: Prentice-Hall.

Leont'ev, A.N. (1981) *Problems of the Development of the Mind*. Moscow: Progress.

Markou, S.N. (1993) *Dyslexia, Left-Handedness, Motion Sickness, Superactivity: Theory, Diagnosis and Treatment with Special Exercises*. Athens: Ellinika Grammata.

Martin, D. (2008) A new paradigm to inform inter-professional learning for integrating speech and language provision into secondary schools: A socio-cultural activity theory approach. *Child Language Teaching and Therapy* 24 (2), 173–192.

Ministry of Education, Lifelong Learning and Religious Affairs (2010) Ministerial Decision 1-3-2010/23519/C2. Exams within schools (Final), written exams during the four month period of students with disability and special educational needs at technical vocational schools, vocational schools. Department of Secondary Education.

MNERA (1983) *Responsibilities of Directors, Directorates and Offices* (PD 340/83). Athens: Ministry of National Education and Religious Affairs.

MNERA (1985) Law 1566/85. Structure and function of primary and secondary education. *Government Gazette* 167 (30 September).

MNERA (1991) *Information Bulletin on Special Education*. Athens: Publishing Association of Textbooks.

MNERA (1994) *Information Bulletin on Special Education: School and Social Inclusion*. Athens: Publishing Association of Textbooks.

MNERA (2000) FEK A'78/14.03.2000. Law 2817/2000. Education of people with special needs and other regulations. Chapter A. Education of people with special educational needs. Article 2.

MNERA (2008) Law 3699/2008. Special education of people with handicap or special educational needs.

MNERA (2009) Within school exams, short time or hourly exams for trimester or four month period of secondary school students with disability and special education needs or specific learning difficulties. Department of Secondary Education.

Nijakowska, J. (2000) Dyslexia – Does it mean anything to a foreign language teacher? In L. Peer. and G. Reid (eds) *Multilingualism, Literacy and Dyslexia: A Challenge for Educators* (pp. 248–256). London: David Fulton Publishers.

Nikolopoulou, A. (1986) School psychology in Greece. *Journal of School Psychology* 24, 325–333.

Pigiaki, P. (1999) The crippled 'pedagogue': Discourses in education and the Greek case. *Educational Review* 51 (1), 55–65.

Reid, G. (2009) *Dyslexia: A Practitioner's Handbook* (4th edn). Chichester: Wiley.

Riddell, S., Brown, S. and Duffield, J. (1994) Conflicts of policies and models: The case of specific learning difficulties. In S. Riddell and S. Brown (eds) *Special Educational Needs Policy in the 1990s* (pp. 113–140). London: Routledge and Kegan Paul.

UNESCO (1994) The Salamanca statement and framework for action on special needs education. World conference in special needs education: Access and Quality. See http://www.unesco.org/education/pdf/SALAMA_E.PDF (accessed June 2013).

Virkkunen, J. and Kuutti, K. (2000) Understanding organizational learning by focusing on 'activity systems'. *Accounting Management and Information Technologies* 10, 291–319.

Vygotsky, L.S. (1987) *Thought and Language*. Cambridge, MA: MIT Press.

7 Multilingual Literacies in Mainstream Classroom Contexts

Jean Conteh

Introduction

This chapter presents a review of research and policy from 2000, related to multilingual literacies and their mediation in mainstream classroom contexts in England. It focuses on learners aged from 5 to 11 years. It includes reference to research into literacy teaching and learning in complementary learning settings and family and community literacy practices, drawing implications for mainstream school learning and constructions of literacy. The main argument is that, in relation to language education and multilingualism, the mediation of multilingual literacies in mainstream classroom contexts is underpinned by 'monolingualising' (Heller, 2007) and 'container' (Martin-Jones, 2007) models of policy and pedagogy. These have a powerful, often negative, impact on the achievement and attainment of multilingual learners and on what are constructed as their learning 'difficulties'.

Current (July 2013) figures for pupils who are categorised as 'multilingual' in mainstream primary and secondary schools in England can be found on the website of the National Association for Language Development in the Curriculum (NALDIC, 2013). They show that there are more than a million such pupils. The term most commonly used in current policy to categorise them is 'EAL' (English as an additional language) learners. Often misinterpreted as referring only to pupils who may also be defined as 'new arrivals' (Department for Education, 2006), 'EAL' is a loose, ill-defined umbrella term for different groups of pupils who bring a vast range of experience and knowledge of languages, cultures, schooling and literacies to their mainstream classrooms. In other discourses, and at times within policy discourses in England, they are labelled 'bilingual' learners. The term 'bilingual' is also a very loose one. A definition that best captures the important links between language and social practice for many EAL learners is that developed by Hall *et al.* (2001) in their work in multilingual schools in Tower Hamlets. They define bilingual pupils as those who:

live in two languages, who have access to, or need to use, two or more languages at home and at school. It does not mean that they have fluency in both languages or that they are competent and literate in both languages. (Hall *et al.*, 2001: 5)

Such pupils are the focus here and I take the term 'multilingual' to be consonant with 'bilingual' for these pupils in this chapter.

After a brief exposition of relevant research paradigms, the chapter is organised in three main sections. The first contextualises the experiences of young multilingual learners in home and community and in mainstream policy and practice contexts in England. Using the theories of researchers such as Cummins (2001), it argues for the positive educational potential of their multilingual experiences. At the same time, it contends that the system fails to recognise both language diversity as a significant and complex factor in learning, and the diverse ways in which home and community experiences can contribute to school learning. The following two sections provide a review of research, policy and practice related to two opposing models of literacies which, it is argued, are currently salient in very different ways for multilingual learners in the primary education system in England. The first is deeply implicated in policy and assessment and so has had a huge influence on practice in mainstream classrooms over recent years. It could be defined as the 'official' literacy. The second has been a growing trend in sociolinguistic and ethnographic research, which is opening out our understanding of the everyday, lived experiences of multilingual learners. It is gradually becoming recognised in limited ways in mainstream practice, though not in policy. The two models are characterised as follows:

- literacy as an orchestration of psychological, language-led decoding and comprehension processes, increasingly constructed in policy and practice as a set of specific, decontextualised skills to be explicitly and discretely taught;
- literacy/ies as sets of socially, culturally and politically contextualised practices that reflect and are constructed through the diversity of learners' experiences in home, school and community.

Research Paradigms

Martin-Jones (2007) provides a historical review of research into bilingualism in education from the 1950s to the present. She defines 'bilingual education' as 'all forms of provision for bilingual learners, including minimal forms of support for learning in and through two languages' (p. 164), but not including programmes for the teaching of English as a second or additional language. The framework and critique that she develops offer a useful starting point from which to consider research relevant to the multilingual learners who are the concern of the present chapter. She suggests (p. 163) that research into bilingual education, almost from its inception, has been largely policy driven and has developed 'a discourse about bilingual education and achievement'. She argues that the type of research that has persistently underpinned this is large-scale, focused on particular cohorts of students, and involves 'the use of standardised tests and the generation of quantitative findings of the type that policy-makers find compelling' (p. 166). Findings from this model of research are frequently used in England to sanction official policies related to literacy teaching (examples are provided below, the next section). But – as we shall see – the picture is not as straightforward, nor as empirically sound, as the methodology and the findings may suggest.

Another important strand of research that Martin-Jones reviews is work in multilingual classrooms of a much more interpretive nature, from ethnomethodological and ethnographic traditions. She suggests that this was 'part of a broader theoretical and methodological turn across the social sciences towards dialogic interaction and social constructionism' in the 1980s (p. 167). Rather than accepting the link between bilingual education and achievement as predetermined and school failure for certain groups as almost inevitable, such research – she argues – begins to 'ask different kinds of questions about the nature of the school experiences for minority students'. Moreover, it develops our understanding of:

> how multilingual resources are managed in different educational contexts, and ... the kinds of discursive routines (bilingual and mono-lingual) that emerge in particular kinds of sociolinguistic conditions, when particular kinds of bilingual arrangements are ushered in with new educational policies. (Martin-Jones, 2007: 170)

Research in this paradigm has usually been conducted in multilingual urban school settings, often following children from home and community to school. It is the focus of the last section of the chapter ('Literacy/ies as sets of social, cultural and politically contextualised practices'). In linking experiences in mainstream classrooms to children's home and community experiences, it contributes to our understanding of how failure in main-stream schooling can be constructed as systemic, rather than the outcome of some kind of imagined 'deficit' in the learner as an individual, which then needs remedial action. Recent research in England (e.g. Blackledge & Creese, 2010) that has followed children into their community-situated, complementary learning settings has opened our eyes to the complex and fascinating ways in which multilingual literacies feature in the lives of young people in England.

As Martin-Jones shows, such research 'arose out of a shared concern with the ways that educational policies and classroom practices contribute to the asymmetries of power between groups with different social and linguistic resources' (p. 171). The development of such a critical approach to research into multilingualism in education has been crucial to our understanding of the ways in which success and failure are systemically constructed, and how:

> in different multilingual contexts, education serves as a means of assigning value to language and literacy resources and, at the same time, as a means of regulating access to them. (Martin-Jones, 2007: 163)

It has led to an understanding both of the ways in which education policies and practices in local contexts related to multilingualism are inevitably and intimately linked to global concerns and of how:

> the necessary educational critique [can] begin to define a future vision for language and literacy education that takes account of increasing local diversity and global connectedness. (Martin-Jones, 2007: 178)

Multilingualism in Practice and Policy in Language Education in Mainstream Primary Schools

Multilingualism in practice

It is the turn of the 21st century. We enter a year 3 classroom in a primary school (for pupils aged between five and nine years) in a multilingual city in the north of England. The setting is typical of many such 'super-diverse' (Vertovec, 2007) areas of Britain and Europe. The fluid and constantly changing populations of such cities have grown into the contemporary, complex and multilayered communities which, Vertovec suggests, require much more subtle and nuanced social policy responses than the 'kind of diversity management strategy that came to be called multiculturalism' (Vertovec, 2007: 1027).

It is lunchtime in our classroom, and three eight-year-old children are sitting round a table talking to a visitor. The children are all British-born, descendants of men who arrived in the city from the Kashmir area of Pakistan 40 or 50 years previously to work in the booming woollen mills. They are talking with the visitor about the books they like to read. One child jumps up, runs across to the class library, quickly finds a book, brings it back to the table and opens it. The three children begin reading aloud together, looking carefully at the book as they do:

01   **3 ch. tog**: (*spelling out*) khargosh ... khargosh
     Visitor: the rabbit ...
     Yasmin: khargosh ... sh ... sh ... *em* ... gha ... gha
     Nahida: ghu ... ghu ...

05 **Yasmin**: khargosh ... gha ...
    Nahida: heh ... spell it out ... gha ...
    Yasmin: what's carrot in Urdu? ... ghajar
    Nahida: ghajar ...
    Anwar: ghajar ...
10 **Yasmin**: ghajar ...
    Nahida: ghajar ... sh ... shawk se kah raha hai ...
    Yasmin: it means ... rabbit is eating ...
    Nahida: the rabbit is eating happily the carrot
    Visitor: the rabbit is happily eating the carrot
15 **Nahida**: eating the carrot
    Yasmin: yeah ... miss

(Conteh, 2003: 46–47)

Yasmin, Nahida and Anwar[1] are all multilingual, and from a minority ethnic, Pakistani-heritage background. All three are successful learners in mainstream school. Conteh (2003: 41–49) traces the ways in which the mediation of their language and learning experiences between home and school underpins their success. As well as English, they speak Punjabi and Urdu. They are also becoming multiliterate (Datta, 2007): all are learning the Koran in Arabic from Muslim teachers, Anwar in his local mosque and Yasmin and Nahida from female teachers who visit their homes. They are also learning to read and write Urdu, their heritage national language. This is done with family members using very formal repetition and rote-learning strategies. While English might be their dominant language, it is clear that other languages have important roles to play in their lives. A study carried out in their home city by Aitsiselmi (2004) reveals the wide and complex array of languages and dialects families such as theirs have at their disposal from their heritage in Pakistan. While English has 'become the main language of communication among siblings, peers and friends for the younger generation', there is a clear consensus among informants of all ages that the heritage languages 'should continue be used' for a range of purposes (Aitsiselmi, 2004: 34). Aitsiselmi suggests that, for his informants, this:

> encapsulate[s] the multiple layers of identities which may be expressed through each of the various languages used for the purposes of spoken or written communication. (Aitsiselmi, 2004: 3)

The book that Yasmin chose from the library, and which the children read with such enthusiasm, was a reading primer in Urdu, of the type that they would be learning from at home. These can be bought throughout Pakistan and India and in 'foreign language' bookshops around the world. In their mainstream classroom, like almost every other Key Stage 2 child in England, the children are learning to read in English – as explained in the next section – through the strategies outlined in the National Curriculum (Department for Education and Employment, 1999) and more closely defined in the Literacy Framework (Department for Education and Skills, 2001). Through tightly organised, fast-paced teacher-led activities, they are being taught to use a range of word-, sentence- and text-focused strategies to decode words and make sense of what they read.

What is interesting about the reading behaviour illustrated in the above transcript is that it shows the children's multiliteracy development in practice. They seem to be transferring the strategies that they have learnt from their literacy lessons in English to their reading of the Urdu text. As they sound out the Urdu syllables and move back and forth across the sentence to construct its meaning, it appears that the strategies they are being taught in order to read in one language are supporting their reading in another. In this way, they are demonstrating something of Cummins' principle of 'interdependence' (Cummins, 2001: 109ff.), part of his model of the 'common underlying proficiency' through which he characterises the language processing of multilingual individuals. Such ideas challenge the commonsense pedagogic notion that, when learning a second language, the learner's first language will in some way interfere and should be avoided.

In the mainstream education system in England, pupils such as Yasmin, Nahida and Anwar are categorised as 'EAL'. They belong to the largest group within the category, sometimes termed 'advanced learners' (Department for Education, 2006). For such pupils, however, as Aitsiselmi (2004) shows, English is really not an 'additional language' at all. It is the one they hear and speak more commonly than those which might be defined as their 'mother tongues'. In their engagement with the reading of the Urdu text, they illustrate clearly Hornberger's model of 'continua of biliteracy' learning as:

> learners' developing communicative competence in socioculturally and sociopolitically contextualised, locally and multiply inclusive, enquiry-based, and dynamically negotiated ways. (Hornberger, 2004: 168)

As Leung et al. (1997: 544) argue, the children are 'actively construct[ing] their own patterns of language use, ethnicity, and social identity', often in 'strong contradiction to the fixed patterns and the reified ethnicities attributed' to them, and – it can be added – in ways that language policies in England do not take account of.

Multilingualism in policy

Multilingualism has been a growing phenomenon in British society for many years, and particularly since the 1970s. Responses in education policy have been contradictory and confused. The forward-looking Bullock report, a full and wide-ranging study of the condition of English teaching in schools entitled *A Language For Life*, made brief allusion to multilingualism, as 'an asset, something to be nurtured' (Department of Education and Science, 1975: 294). It acknowledged both its local and national benefits, for 'the children and their families, and also society as a whole' (p. 293). Ten years later, following a national period of political and social unrest, the Swann report, *Education For All* (Department of Education and Science, 1985) promoted an assimilationist 'equal access' ideology in which educational provision needed, above all, to achieve equality of opportunity and en-titlement for everyone. One of its key recommendations, the ending of local authority provision for the teaching of so-called 'community languages', resulted in the separation of mainstream school and community in terms of provision for language learning, and the termination of research projects to investigate the links between mother tongue and English in children's learning. The wider implications of this were clearly not foreseen at the time, but have emerged since through research studies such as that by Martin-Jones and Saxena (1995, 1996). Swann also strongly encouraged the replacing of provision for the learning of English for new arrivals in separate language centres or special classes within school with mainstream provision. Coincidentally, the so-called Calderdale report (Commission for Racial Equality, 1986) concluded that the practice of withdrawal for pupils new to English was 'racist' (Gravelle, 1996: 73). This led to a rush nationally to close down language centres and introduce 'language support teachers' to meet the needs of new arrivals in mainstream settings (Gravelle, 1996: 6–7).

Official responses in primary education policy in England in relation to curriculum and assessment for multilingual pupils have been similarly inconsistent. The tensions between 'diversity' and 'inclusion' are well documented (Ainscow *et al.*, 2007; Conteh, 2006). Safford (2003: 8) argues that we have 'conflicting policy paradigms' in relation to multilingualism and assessment. She suggests that 'the celebration of ethnic and linguistic diversity' – often mediated in curriculum guidance through the 'multi-cultural' ideology of 'sari, samosas and steel bands' (Troyna & Williams, 1986: 24) – sits uncomfortably alongside the 'universal model of language development and assessment' which is embedded in the system. How, she asks, 'if we have a single statutory model of language learning and assess-ment', can diversity 'truly influence educational provision'? These issues are further discussed below. The contradictions are woven through the National Curriculum, introduced in 1988. Its 'equality of opportunity' aims led to a re-assertion of entitlement to standard English (Cameron & Bourne, 1988) and an overall 'monolingualising' (Heller, 2007) ethos. This meant that community languages might be constructed in accompanying guidance as a 'rich resource' (National Curriculum Council, 1991: 1), but only until such time as children were confident enough in English to do without them – in a clear manifestation of Martin-Jones's 'container' (2007: 166) approach to bilingual education.

A complex system of national assessment practices was quickly instituted alongside the curriculum. Despite the work of the 'multicultural task group' (Tomlinson, 1993: 21), which developed detailed suggestions for a curriculum for bilingual pupils, the National Curriculum took no account of the diversity of ways in which young multilingual learners' language capacities and knowledge needed to be assessed differently from their 'monolingual' peers. Gregory's critique of the curriculum and its 'equal opportunities' ideology posed the question, 'Could it be that, paradoxically, provision of the same curriculum for all might actually prevent some children from gaining access to it?' (Gregory, 1994: 151). She shows how the National Curriculum and its assessment frameworks take virtually no account of what was known at the time – and has been reinforced since – from research about successful second language learning, nor from international comparisons of provision for multilingual learners.

The Swann report's 'equal opportunities' agenda led to another development which, paradoxically, introduced bilingual adults into multilingual classrooms at the same time as contributing to the closing down of multilingual opportunities for learning. Following Swann's recommendation, bilingual support assistants quickly became common and in some multilingual schools they now outnumber qualified teachers. Swann's description of their role captures the ways in which, within the endeavour of becoming a successful pupil in the mainstream system in England, multilingualism is seen as transitional at best. The assistant is characterised as a 'bilingual resource' who provides:

> a degree of continuity between the home and school environment by offering psychological and social support for the child, as well as being able to explain simple educational concepts in a child's mother tongue, if the need arises, but always working within the mainstream classroom and alongside the class teacher. (Department of Education and Science, 1985: 407–408)

This is in no way to undervalue the important roles that many bilingual support assistants play, often beyond their professional rewards and recognition (Martin-Jones & Saxena, 2003). But it reflects the status of bilingualism in the system generally and the model of 'EAL' learners as simply being those children who are 'new arrivals', needing support for a few weeks or months until they can understand English. Bourne argues that professional discourses in English primary classrooms are historically strongly hierarchical, leading to the construction of pedagogies that view language diversity as 'problems' (Bourne, 2001: 262). With the growth in numbers of bilingual support assistants and other kinds of teaching assistants, discourses in primary classrooms have become mediated in increasingly asymmetrical ways. Moreover, despite strenuous efforts by government agencies, the numbers of qualified bilingual teachers in primary schools in England remain persistently low (Conteh, 2007: 462) and so the most common model is of a monolingual teacher directing the work of a bilingual assistant. It is not surprising, then, that 'subtractive bilingualism' (Cummins, 2001: 106) prevails in primary schools in England.

In terms of curriculum and pedagogic guidance, generic principles for teachers are contained in the statement on inclusion, 'Including all learners', which prefaces the 2000 version of the National Curriculum (Department for Education and Employment, 1999: 30–34). The contradictions are clear, not just in the text itself, but in its intentions. A statement of inclusion seems to beg the question of how the learners referred to came to be excluded in the first place. It implies a model of an 'idealised primary pupil' with a notional set of qualities that enables her or him to perform to a fixed and absolute standard of success. It is clear from the statement that pupils 'from diverse linguistic backgrounds' do not conform to such an ideal. First of all, teachers need to 'take specific action' (presumably beyond the actions they are expected to take in their normal roles as teachers) to respond to their 'diverse needs'. The list of possible actions is a somewhat odd mix, including 'securing their motivation and concentration' and 'providing equality of opportunity'. Nowhere in the list is there specific reference to language pedagogy, nor to the possibility that teachers may need to consider in their planning and teaching the distinctive language and cultural experiences that their multilingual pupils may bring to their learning. The statement goes on – more worryingly – to include pupils 'who are learning English as an additional language' in the category of those with 'potential barriers' to their learning. This section does make passing reference to their 'skills in other languages', but does not provide any clues as to how these could be marshalled as a resource for their learning of English, nor to how the children's multilingualism could be a benefit in their learning more generally.

Construction of the 'Official' Literacy

Literacy in the National Curriculum and the National Literacy Strategy

English, not literacy, is defined as a subject within the 1988 National Curriculum, and its structure and content have largely been retained through to the curriculum's current manifestation (Department for Education and Employment, 1999). This remains the national statutory requirement for school provision, despite the plethora of advice and guidance materials that have since been introduced, particularly for primary schools. English as a subject is packaged into three programmes of study: listening and speaking, reading, and writing. There is one set of each for Key Stage 1 (KS1) (pupils aged 5–7 years) and Key Stage 2 (KS2) (pupils aged 7–11 years). In the KS1 programme of study for reading, En2 (Department for Education and Employment, 1999: 18), there is a clear statement of 'the range of strategies' that pupils need to be taught to use in order to 'read with fluency, accuracy, understanding and enjoyment'. These are:

- phonemic awareness and phonic knowledge;
- word recognition and graphic knowledge;
- grammatical awareness;
- contextual understanding.

Each is amplified by a set of specific but broadly defined actions (which could perhaps be categorised as skills) which pupils are expected to be able to perform, ranging from 'identify syllables in words' to 'understand how word order affects meaning'. The same set of four 'reading strategies' is prescribed for KS2 (Department for Education and Employment, 1999: 25). But here 'enjoyment' is not listed as an element of reading and the lists of specific 'skills' from KS1 are not included. Alongside this, the programmes of study for writing (pp. 20–21, 28–30) have the same kind of skills-related discourse in relation to spelling and handwriting, but a more holistic discourse in relation to the compositional elements of writing. In terms of content, the curriculum is sparse, but there is brief allusion to the need to provide resources which might be seen to reflect multilingualism or language diversity; the KS1 programme of study makes reference to 'stories and poems from a range of cultures' (p. 19) and at KS2 there is reference to 'texts drawn from a variety of cultures and traditions' (p. 26).

Despite the introduction of the National Curriculum, in the 1990s in England there was a growing, but not empirically well grounded, concern about standards in education. A focus of this was the teaching of reading, purportedly supported with evidence from the recently introduced national testing regimes for 7- and 11-year-olds (the TASKS or SATs), various reports from the schools Inspectorate and the politically popular 'school improvement' discourses informed by large-scale, survey-type research. Beard (1999: 16–26) provides an overview. Such evidence, which, as Beard demonstrates, largely focuses on pupils from 'disadvantaged' backgrounds, has been extensively critiqued and consistently found wanting (e.g. Goldstein & Mortimore, 2011; Mortimore & Goldstein, 1996). Large-scale surveys of SATs results, particularly of primary schools, where the numbers of pupils taking the tests are often insufficient to demonstrate statistical significance, are commonly taken as watertight evidence for poor-quality teaching or other failures within the system, despite the fact that they often suffer from major methodological flaws. In terms of the teaching of reading, they led, among other outcomes, to the introduction of the National Literacy Project (NLP) (1997) in 15 local education authorities (LEAs) (Beard, 1999: 27).

Beard notes (p. 29) that nearly all the 250 schools involved were in urban, disadvantaged areas. The project had the following aims, among others:

- to improve standards of literacy in participating primary schools, in line with national expectations;
- to provide detailed support to schools and teachers through a structured programme and consultancy support;
- through the national network, to develop detailed, practical guidance on teaching methods and activities, and to disseminate these to the project schools.

Following the change of government in 1997, the NLP rapidly meta-morphosised into the National Literacy Strategy (NLS). This ushered in a huge and unprecedented focus on literacy as a key preoccupation in primary education. In 2001, a new framework for teaching, with the 'Literacy Hour' at its centre, was introduced (Department for Education and Skills, 2001). This was a file of materials that provided teachers with planning pro formas and detailed learning objectives. Though not statutory, it came with a massive panoply of training and resourcing, media coverage, inspection accountability and political pressure.

The two main models of literacy that underpinned the Literacy Hour were: first, the 'searchlights' model of reading; and second, the 'genre' approach to teaching about texts. The searchlights model (see Figure 7.1) characterises the reading process as involving four 'sources of knowledge' – called 'searchlights' – which the reader 'turns on' to the text, as appropriate, to 'illuminate' meaning. The inclusion in the file of learning objectives makes it clear that 'successful readers use as many of these strategies as possible' (p. 3), but that phonics should predominate. These four strategies clearly align with the four 'strategies' that largely constitute reading in the National Curriculum. But the Literacy Hour framework, with its termly lists of learning objectives at word, sentence and text level, goes much further to construe the processes of reading as a set of skills, all of which have to be taught explicitly. This skills-based approach to teaching sits alongside a genre-based model of texts, which can clearly be discerned in many of the text-level learning objectives. Based on Hallidayan systemic functional grammar principles (Derewianka, 1990), this model offers powerful pedagogic possibilities, different from a skills-based one, in its focus on authentic language and on the multimodality of texts. It replaces conventional, prescriptive notions of grammar with a functional model of grammar as a set of tools with which speakers or writers achieve their com-municative purposes.

Such an approach to literacy pedagogy has potential for recognising and valuing the diversity of language resources which learners generally, and multilingual learners in particular, bring to their classrooms, succinctly represented by Garcia (2009) as:

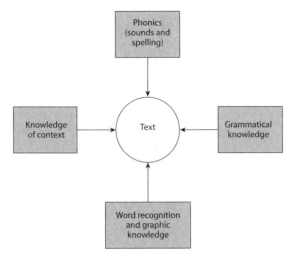

Figure 7.1 The searchlights model of reading underpinning the Literacy Hour

the multiplicity of individual and group repertoires, and the varied communicative purposes for which groups use different spoken, signed and written languages. (Garcia, 2009: 339)

Drawing on the work of the New London group (Cope & Kalantzis, 2000), Garcia goes on (2009: 352) to define four principles for 'meaningful pedagogy' that promote multiliteracy, and which have clear parallels with the genre-based approach in the Literacy Hour framework. Work supported by the National Association for Language Development in the Curriculum (2010) has gone some way to explore the potential of the functional approach for multilingual learners. Unfortunately, this potential is not clearly articulated in the Literacy Hour framework. Moreover, the framework was introduced in a rushed and prescriptive way, swiftly followed by a plethora of commercial material from publishers keen to capitalise on its demands – for example the '100 Literacy Framework Lessons' (Scholastic, 2011), currently available to match the renewed primary framework. This meant that, by and large, mainstream teachers did not develop the knowledge about language, nor the professional confidence, to take ownership of the principles underpinning genre-based teaching.

Literacy pedagogy developed in multilingual and multicultural contexts – such as Holdaway's (1979) approaches, from New Zealand, to using big books and shared reading – figures prominently in the Literacy Hour. But, ironically, multilingualism was not seen as a priority, nor even an aspect of children's experience that teachers needed to seriously consider.

Beard's *post hoc* review of research underpinning the strategy (Beard, 1999) makes no mention whatsoever of multilingualism or language diversity. Neither, in its first manifestation, did the Literacy Hour file. But its arrival in schools in 2001 was hastily followed by the distribution of 'Section 4', a pack of materials designed to be slotted into the back of the file. This provided 'additional guidance' for a miscellaneous list of pupils in a range of circumstances: mixed-year classes, small schools, reception-aged children, children speaking (*sic*) English as an additional language and children with special educational needs. It comprises 21 pages, with seven pages devoted to EAL learners. There is some reference to the importance of teachers having 'information about pupils' educational history and their literacy skills in another language' (p. 110) and also to 'the place of languages other than English' (p. 111) in the learning of English literacy. But the ultimate goal is clear: by the end of KS2, multilingual learners need to perform in just the same ways as their 'monolingual' peers. Small-scale, qualitative research from the years immediately following the introduction of the Literacy Hour (e.g. Moss, 2002; Wallace, 2005) shows how it redefined what counted as literacy in school. Through evidence from conversations with children, Wallace argues that the skills-based, reductive model of literacy mediated in the Literacy Hour 'may fail to do justice to the full range of children's cultural and cognitive resources, especially when children are not from mainstream social groups' (Wallace, 2005: 337).

A watershed in literacy practice and assessment – The question of phonics

The concern about standards was not calmed by the imposition of the Literacy Hour framework, nor its renewed framework, introduced online in 2006 and in 2011 archived by a new government. As Goouch and Lambirth (2008: 2) show, the concern reached the level of a 'panic' that centred on the 'long tail of under-achievement' in the system in England. These are the pupils considered to have failed to have met the required standards, inevitably mostly from low-income families, and many of them EAL learners. The scene was set for the publication of the so-called 'independent' Rose review of early reading (Department for Education and Skills, 2006), a watershed in policy and practice in relation to literacy in primary education in England. Heavily based on psychological research into the 'cognitive processes involved in reading', the review reached the conclusion that the searchlights model had been superseded by research findings and needed to be modified:

> We think that further progress towards the goal of using evidence derived from psychological research to inform teaching practice will be better achieved if the searchlights model is now reconstructed into the two

components of reading (word recognition, language comprehension) that are present but confounded within it. (Department for Education and Skills, 200: 75)

And so, the 'simple view' of reading was given official sanction, with systematic synthetic phonics (SSP) enshrined as the universal panacea to the problem of how to teach young learners to read. Torgerson *et al.* (2006: 19–20) trace the trajectory of SSP from official concern with underachievement to embedding in classroom practice. The official pressure in England to move primary classroom practice in early literacy towards SSP is, arguably, currently felt most strongly in initial teacher education (e.g. Training and Development Agency for Schools, 2011). In this context, discourses of deficit related to multilingual learners are reinforced in the 33 standards of professional knowledge, understanding and skills currently required by all newly qualified teachers (NQTs) (Training and Development Agency for Schools, 2007), currently under review. In only one, 'Q19', is 'EAL' explicitly mentioned, linked inextricably with 'SEN' (special educational need) and pupils with 'disabilities', so reinforcing the assumption that 'EAL' relates only to pupils who are somehow in deficit and have limited knowledge of English. This, of course, has huge implications for primary pedagogy. The expectation that pupils 'learning EAL' will find things difficult is also clear in the Rose review (e.g. p. 52, para. 170). Aspect 1, about 'best practice', includes a section about 'English as an additional language' (pp. 23–25, paras 64–71), which repeats the same bland, general advice found elsewhere in Literacy Strategy documentation (Department for Education and Skills, 2001). It seems to imply that the introduction of a 'commercial phonics scheme' is the route to success for schools with high proportions of EAL learners. The promises of such schemes are seductive to teachers. And, as Hall (2006: 20) reminds us, there are huge financial rewards awaiting 'anyone who invents the best scheme or programme' for teaching phonics.

The Rose review's claim that 'synthetic phonics offers the vast majority of beginners the best route to becoming skilled readers' (p. 19) is based largely on the so-called 'Clackmannanshire studies' (Johnston & Watson, 2004, 2005). Researchers in early literacy in England, from both psychological and pedagogic arenas, have almost unanimously questioned the validity of the studies, for a variety of reasons (e.g. Goswami, pp. 136–139, and Wyse, pp. 125–126, both in Goouch & Lambirth, 2008). Johnston and Watson's conclusions have also been called into question in measured ways in Torgerson *et al.*'s systematic review of randomised controlled trials into the role of SSP in literacy instruction (Torgerson *et al.*, 2006: 20, 55–56). Their key findings about the effect of phonics on reading (p. 8) need to be carefully considered. Perhaps their subtleties were missed in the rush to find a simple solution to the problem of teaching children to read and for addressing the 'long tail of underachievement':

- Systematic phonics instruction within a broad literacy curriculum was found to have a statistically significant positive effect on reading *accuracy*.
- There was no statistically significant difference between the effectiveness of systematic phonics instruction for reading accuracy for normally developing children and for children at risk of reading failure.
- The weight of evidence for both these findings was moderate (there were 12 randomised controlled trials included in the analysis).
- Both of these findings provided some support for those of a systematic review published in the United States in 2001 (Ehri *et al.*, 2001).
- An analysis of the effect of systematic phonics instruction on reading *comprehension* was based on weak weight of evidence (only four randomised controlled trials were found) and failed to find the statistically significant positive difference which was found in the previous review.

Hall (2006: 12) suggests that researchers like Johnston and Watson were 'asking the wrong research question', and were not paying attention to the ways that young literacy learners actually develop their understandings of reading and engage with the whole phenomenon of literacy, an idea that is supported by qualitative research into children's learning. She contextualises her critique in a discussion of the 'full dimensions' of literacy for young learners, as well as evidence from research about how young learners themselves approach the task of learning to read. The same approach is taken by Gregory, who reminds us of the prevailing 'monolingualism' of mainstream school practices by pointing out how references to 'language' in the Rose review are synonymous with 'English' (Gregory, 2008: 111). She provides a wealth of qualitative evidence about how young multilingual learners engage with the literacies that they encounter in their schools, homes and communities. She demonstrates the ways in which their experiences of different languages and scripts contribute to their metalinguistic awareness (p. 107), illustrating the 'syncretism' of their literacy learning in similar ways to Yasmin, Nahida and Anwar in their engagement with the text in Urdu presented above. Gregory's discussion of the role of phonics in reading for multilingual learners includes the engaging account of Saida, a young child recently arrived from Bangladesh. Saida could accurately decode words in an English reading scheme book, without comprehending what she had 'read' (p. 123), in the same way as she could decode the Arabic she was learning in the mosque. Luckily, her teacher had the imagination to think of ways to use her pupil's knowledge of the sounds of the letters as a resource to lead her into reading for meaning. Gregory concludes that knowledge of sound–symbol correspondences in any language provides the young multilingual learner with an initial advantage, but that the move to meaningful engagement with text needs to be quickly made.

Literacy/ies as Sets of Social, Cultural and Politically Contextualised Practices

In her survey of research into bilingual education, Martin-Jones (2007: 167–168) points out 'the explanatory limits of the large scale survey' and the growing interest 'in the negotiation of meaning in and through inter-action' which led to the qualitative, interpretative kind of research which is the focus of this section of the chapter. The intention is to provide starting points for considering constructions of literacy that are different from the 'official' model that predominates in mainstream classrooms, and which may more accurately reflect the experiences of multilingual learners in England. Through this, it becomes possible to contest the increasingly inevitable links made between multilingualism and learning difficulties. Recent years have seen an exponential growth of research in literacy in diverse contexts, within methodological paradigms such as ethnographies of literacy (Baynham, 2004), Syncretic Literacy Studies (Gregory *et al.*, 2004), New Literacy Studies (Pahl & Rowsell, 2005; Street, 1984) and eth-nographies of multilingualism (Blackledge & Creese, 2010). All are grounded in sociocultural models of learning which, as Gregory *et al.* (2004: 7) argue, have the overarching goal of putting 'culture in the middle' and understand-ing 'the nature of the culture–cognition link in everyday life', in line with Vygotskyan thinking. Common goals related to literacy through all this work are the 're-evaluation of what counts as literacy' and the relating of 'situated literacy activity to macro relations of social power and dominance' (Baynham, 2004: 286).

Baynham's overview of ethnographies of literacy points to the 'classic, first-generation studies' of Scribner and Cole (1981), Heath (1983) and Street (1984), all of which provide rich evidence of community-based practices in literacy. Linking Sierra Leone, Liberia, the south-eastern United States and Iran, these studies all open perceptions of what literacy entails. They have in common the use of anthropological principles to document the full range of literacy practices in the communities they studied, whether the 'indigenous scripts' devised by Vai people in west Africa, the 'literacy events' that parents engaged in with their children in African-American and white working-class families in the Carolinas or the 'maktab' and 'commercial' literacies of 1970s Iran. Common to all of these socially situated literacy practices is the fact that they slip under the radar of the 'official' literacies mediated by govern-ment literacy education policy in their respective national contexts.

Gregory *et al.*'s contribution to our understanding of literacies is a range of small-scale, largely longitudinal ethnographic studies of how 'young children learn to become members of different cultural practices, involving different languages, literacies, materials and ways of interacting together' (p. 20). A key conclusion the authors draw is that young children become literate through interaction with a diverse range of teachers – such as siblings, grandparents and other family members – in home, school and community, many of them 'invisible' to the mainstream education system. They demonstrate how young learners have the capacity to mediate and indeed actively synthesise their understandings of literacy from these rich 'funds of knowledge' (Gonzalez et al., 2005) in order to take ownership of their own learning. This approach to researching and theorising learning, particularly the practitioner-led models of research into community practices that Gonzalez et al. illustrate (2005: 18–19) helps to reveal the extent and quality of home and community knowledge available to pupils.

Pahl and Rowsell (2005) declare from the outset that their aim is to open out pedagogic possibilities by encouraging teachers to 'come to literacy with a different premise' (p. 1) from the 'drill and skill-based' model of literacy emphasised internationally by government programmes. Taking the New Literacy model, developed by Street (1984) and others, of literacies as social practices embedded in the ideologies and power structures of societies, they argue for a multimodal and multiliterate approach to understanding literacy and developing pedagogy. Based on ethnographic studies which feature closely observed analyses of children's engagements with texts in different media, they use Kress's (1997, 2003) theories of multimodality to show how children's engagements with literacy are much wider and more complex than 'official' models encompass. In a chapter which focuses on the kinds of multilingual classrooms which have been the central concern of this chapter, Pahl and Rowsell argue for the need to understand equally both 'the relationship between multimodality and globalization' and 'how the multimodal and the global function within local contexts' in order to play to the strengths of, and address the needs of, multilingual learners in mainstream classrooms (Pahl & Rowsell, 2005: 76).

The notion of identity figures strongly in Pahl and Rowsell's ideas about multilingual learning and pedagogy, and it is also central in the growing body of research into multilingual learners' experiences in complementary (also known as supplementary) learning settings. Complementary schools have been on the margins of educational policy since the publication of the Swann report, but they are increasingly becoming recognised as 'safe spaces' in which young multilingual learners can explore their identities (Conteh & Brock, 2010). Garcia (2009: 233–234) provides a brief overview of community-based provision for bilingual education around the world. Conteh et al. (2007: 1–19) provide a critical historical review of research and policy related to complementary schooling in Britain, as well as examples of such provision. Lytra and Martin (2010) bring together research on complementary schools in Britain, examining their language and literacy practices and their implications for policy and mainstream pedagogy. Blackledge and Creese's (2010) study of multilingual education has at its core the longitudinal, linguistic ethnographic studies they undertook as part of a team which carried out case studies in Gujarati, Turkish, Mandarin, Cantonese and Bengali complementary schools in different multilingual cities in England in 2006–07 (pp. 10–11). Their research methodology allowed them to engage with the ways in which language practices are socially and politically situated, to explore the subjectivities and viewpoints of all participants, particularly the bilingual teachers, to recognise the ways in which global factors intersect with and impact on the local, and to critique the 'monolingual mindset' ideologies which prevail in education policy in England.

The closing chapters of Blackledge and Creese invite us to view complementary schools on a wider scale, and so lead to fuller consideration of some of the educational, ideological and political strands woven through the book. The authors present an account of the history of the 'oppositional discourse' surrounding the concept of nationhood, and then demonstrate through examples how this is played out in 'the local' (Blackledge & Creese, 2010: 183). Similarly, as part of the Multiliteracies Project (Cope & Kalantzis, 2000), Lo Bianco (2000: 99) provides a rich set of examples of 'script meaning making' from Vietnam, Japan, Australia and England, which demonstrate the tensions between 'the complex literacy awareness and practices' of young people around the world and educational policy which 'define[s] the literacies and languages of immigrant minority and indigenous students as defective by assessment against established norms'. This results, he argues, in 'squandered bilingualism' (Lo Bianco, 2000: 100) through its inability 'to comprehend the intellectualization of a potential bilingual skill'. As the growing body of evidence from the research surveyed in this section – and, indeed, the chapter as a whole – shows, these are the issues which must be addressed in future research in order for us to understand fully the links between multilingualism, achievement and learning 'difficulties'. Ways need to be found to link this with policy constructions and mediations that lead to classroom pedagogies which benefit from the multilingual resources of our pupils, affording the 'collaborative creation of power' between teacher and pupil which Cummins (2001) predicts will transform classroom practice and the potential for success.

Note

1   These are pseudonyms for children who took part in a small-scale, ethnographic study of 'successful' bilingual pupils at KS2 in a mainstream school (Conteh, 2003).

References

Ainscow, M., Conteh, J., Dyson, A. and Gallanaugh, F. (2007) *Children in Primary Education: Demography, Culture, Diversity and Inclusion* (Primary Review Research Survey 5/1). Cambridge: University of Cambridge Faculty of Education. See http://arrts.gtcni. org.uk/gtcni/bitstream/2428/26673/1/Primary_Review_5-1_report_Demography-culture-diversity-inclusion_071214.pdf (accessed January 2012).

Aitsiselmi, F. (2004) *Linguistic Diversity and the Use of English in the Home Environment: A Bradford Case Study.* Department of Languages and European Studies, School of Social and International Studies, University of Bradford.

Baynham, M. (2004) Ethnographies of literacy: Introduction. *Language and Education* 18 (4), 285–290.

Beard, R. (1999) *National Literacy Strategy: Review of Research and Other Related Evidence* London: Department for Education and Employment.

Blackledge, A. and Creese, A. (2010) *Multilingualism: Critical Perspectives.* London: Continuum.

Bourne, J. (2001) Doing 'what comes naturally': How the discourses and routines of teachers' practice constrain opportunities for bilingual support in UK primary schools, *Language and Education* 15 (4), 250–268.

Cameron, D. and Bourne, J. (1988) No common ground: Kingman, grammar and nation. *Language and Education* 2 (3), 147–160.

Commission for Racial Equality (CRE) (1986) *Teaching English as a Second Language, Report of a Formal Investigation in Calderdale LEA.* London: CRE.

Conteh, J. (2003) *Succeeding in Diversity: Culture, Language and Learning in Primary Classrooms.* Stoke-on-Trent: Trentham Books.

Conteh, J. (2006) Widening the inclusion agenda: Policy, practice and language diversity in the primary curriculum. In R. Webb (ed.) *Changing Teaching and Learning in the Primary School* (pp. 128–138). Buckingham: Open University Press.

Conteh, J. (2007) Opening doors to success in multilingual classrooms: Bilingualism, codeswitching and the professional identities of 'ethnic minority' primary teachers. *Language and Education* 21 (6), 457–472.

Conteh, J. and Brock, A. (2010) Safe spaces? Sites of bilingualism for young learners in home, school and community. *International Journal of Bilingual Education and Bilingualism* 14 (3), 347–360.

Conteh, J., Martin, P. and Helavaara Robertson, L. (eds) (2007) *Multilingual Learning Stories in Schools and Communities in Britain.* Stoke-on-Trent: Trentham Books.

Cope, B. and Kalantzis, M. (eds) (2000) *Multiliteracies: Literacy Learning and the Design of Social Futures.* London: Routledge.

Cummins, J. (2001) *Negotiating Identities: Education for Empowerment in a Diverse Society* (2nd edn). Ontario, CA: California Association for Bilingual Education.

Datta, M. (ed.) (2007) *Bilinguality and Literacy: Principles and Practice* (2nd edn). London: Continuum.

Department of Education and Science (DES) (1975) *A Language for Life* (Bullock report). London: HMSO.

Department of Education and Science (DES) (1985) *Education For All – The Report of the Committee of Inquiry into the Education of Children from Ethnic Minority Groups* (Swann report). London: HMSO.

Department for Education (DfE) (2006) *New Arrivals Excellence Programme (NAEP).* See http://webarchive.nationalarchives.gov.uk/20110202093118/http://nationalstrategies.standards.dcsf.gov.uk/node/152188 (accessed January 2012).

Department for Education and Employment (DfEE) (1999) *The National Curriculum for England.* See http://curriculum.qcda.gov.uk/key-stages-1-and-2/subjects/english/keystage1/index.aspx (accessed January 2012).

Department for Education and Skills (DfES) (2001) *The National Literacy Strategy: Framework for Teaching* (DfES 0500/2001).

Department for Education and Skills (DfES) (2006) *Independent Review of the Teaching of Early Reading: Final Report* (the Rose review). London: HMSO.

Derewianka, B. (1990) *Exploring How Texts Work.* Sydney: Primary English Teaching Association.

Ehri, L.C., Nunes, S.R., Stahl, S.A. and Willows, D.M. (2001) Systematic phonics instruction helps students learn to read: Evidence from the National Reading Panel's meta-analysis. *Review of Educational Research* 71 (3), 393–447.

Garcia, O. (2009) *Bilingual Education in the 21st Century: A Global Perspective.* Oxford: Wiley-Blackwell.

Goldstein, H. and Mortimore, P. (2011) Misinterpreting KS1 test scores. See http://www.bristol.ac.uk/cmm/team/hg/ks1-crit.html (accessed January 2012).

Gonzalez, N., Moll, L. and Amanti, C. (eds.) (2005) *Funds of Knowledge: Theorizing Practices in Households, Communities and Classrooms.* New York: Routledge.

Goouch, K. and Lambirth, A. (eds) (2008) *Understanding Phonics and the Teaching of Reading: Critical Perspectives.* New York: McGraw Hill/Open University Press.

Gravelle, M. (1996) *Supporting Bilingual Learners in Schools.* Stoke-on-Trent: Trentham.

Gregory, E. (1994) The National Curriculum and non-native speakers of English. In G.V. Blenkin and A.V. Kelly (eds) *The National Curriculum and Early Learning* (pp. 148–171). London: Paul Chapman.

Gregory, E. (2008) *Learning to Read in a New Language: Making Sense of Words and Worlds* (2nd edn). London: Sage.

Gregory, E., Long, S. and Volk, D. (eds) (2004) *Many Pathways to Literacy: Young Children Learning with Siblings, Grandparents, Peers and Communities.* London: Routledge.

Hall, D., Griffiths, D., Haslam, L. and Wilkin, Y. (2001) *Assessing the Needs of Bilingual Pupils: Living in Two Languages* (2nd edn). London: David Fulton.

Hall, K. (2006) How children learn to read and how phonics helps. In M. Lewis and S. Ellis (eds) *Phonics: Practice, Research and Policy* (pp. 9–22). Paul Chapman/UKLA.

Heath, S.B. (1983) *Ways With Words: Life and Work in Communities and Classrooms.* Cambridge: Cambridge University Press.

Heller, M. (ed.) (2007) *Bilingualism: A Social Approach.* London: Palgrave Macmillan.

Holdaway, D. (1979) *The Foundations of Literacy.* Sydney: Ashton Scholastic.

Hornberger, N.H. (2004) The continua of biliteracy and the bilingual educator: Educational linguistics in practice. *International Journal of Bilingual Education and Bilingualism* 7 (2, 3), 155–171.

Johnston, R.S. and Watson, J.E. (2004) Accelerating the development of reading, spelling and phonemic awareness skills in initial readers. *Reading and Writing: An Interdisciplinary Journal* 17 (4), 327–357.

Johnston, R.S. and Watson, J.E. (2005) *The Effects of Synthetic Phonics Teaching on Reading and Spelling Attainment: A Seven Year Longitudinal Study.* See http://www.scotland.gov.uk/Publications/2005/02/20688/52449 (accessed January 2012).

Kress, G. (1997) *Before Writing: Rethinking the Paths to Literacy.* London: Routledge.

Kress, G. (2003) *Literacy in the New Media Age.* London: Routledge.

Leung, C., Harris, R. and Rampton, B. (1997) The idealised native speaker, reified ethnicities, and classroom realities. *TESOL Quarterly* 31 (3), 543–560.

Lo Bianco, J. (2000) Multiliteracies and multilingualism. In B. Cope and M. Kalantzis (eds) *Multiliteracies: Literacy Learning and the Design of Social Futures* (pp. 92–105). London: Routledge.

Lytra, V. and Martin, P. (eds) (2010) *Sites of Multilingualism: Complementary Schools in Britain Today.* Stoke-on-Trent: Trentham Books.

Martin-Jones, M. (2007) Bilingualism, education and the regulation of access to language resources. In M. Heller (ed.) *Bilingualism: A Social Approach* (pp. 161–181). London: Palgrave Macmillan.

Martin-Jones, M. and Saxena, M. (1995) Supporting or containing bilingualism? Policies, power asymmetries and pedagogic practices in mainstream primary schools. In J. Tollefson (ed.) *Power and Inequality in Language Education* (pp. 73–90). Cambridge: Cambridge University Press.

Martin-Jones, M. and Saxena, M. (1996) Turn-taking, power asymmetries, and the positioning of bilingual participants in classroom discourse. *Linguistics and Education* 8 (1), 105–123.

Martin-Jones, M. and Saxena, M. (2003) Bilingual resources and 'funds of knowledge' for teaching and learning in multi-ethnic classrooms in Britain. *International Journal of Bilingual Education and Bilingualism* 6 (3, 4), 267–281.

Mortimore, P. and Goldstein, H. (1996) *The Teaching of Reading in 45 Inner London Secondary Schools: A Critical Examination Offsets Research*. London: Institute of Education.

Moss, G. (2002) Literacy and pedagogy in flux: Constructing the object of study from a Bernsteinian perspective. *British Journal of Sociology of Education* 23 (4), 549–558.

National Association for Language Development in the Curriculum (NALDIC) (2010) *Language Support in EAL Contexts: Why Systemic Functional Linguistics?* (Special issue of *NALDIC Quarterly on Functional Grammar*). See http://oro.open.ac.uk/25026/1/NaldicSFL.pdf (accessed January 2012).

National Association for Language Development in the Curriculum (NALDIC) (2013) The latest EAL facts and figures. See http://www.naldic.org.uk/research-and-information/eal-statistics (accessed July 2013).

National Curriculum Council (NCC) (1991) *Linguistic Diversity and the National Curriculum* (Circular Number 11, March). York: National Curriculum Council.

Pahl, K. and Rowsell, J. (2005) *Literacy and Education: Understanding the New Literacy Studies in the Classroom*. London: Paul Chapman.

Safford, K. (2003) *Teachers and Pupils in the Big Picture: Seeing Real Children in Routinised Assessment*. Watford: National Association for Language Development in the Curriculum (NALDIC).

Scholastic (2011) *100 Literacy Framework Lessons: Complete Set*. See http://shop.scholastic.co.uk/products/1513 (accessed January 2012).

Scribner, S. and Cole, M. (1981) *The Psychology of Literacy*. Cambridge, MA: Harvard University Press.

Street, B. (1984) *Literacy in Theory and Practice*. Cambridge: Cambridge University Press.

Tomlinson, S. (1993) The multicultural task group: The group that never was. In A. King and M. Reis (eds) *The Multicultural Dimension of the National Curriculum* (pp. 21–31). London: Falmer Press.

Torgerson, C., Brooks, G. and Hall, J. (2006) *A Systematic Review of the Research Literature on the Use of Phonics in the Teaching of Reading and Spelling* (Report RR711). Sheffield: DfES/University of Sheffield.

Training and Development Agency for Schools (TDA) (2007) *Professional Standards for Teachers*. See http://www.tda.gov.uk/teacher/developing-career/professional-standards-guidance/professional-standards.aspx (accessed January 2012).

Training and Development Agency for Schools (TDA) (2011) *Training and Development Agency for Schools Primary Priorities for Literacy and Mathematics ITT: Leading Partners in Literacy and Mathematics Programme* (call for proposals to ITT providers, July).

Troyna, B. and Williams, J. (1986) *Racism, Education and the State*. London: Croom Helm.

Vertovec, S. (2007) Super-diversity and its implication. *Ethnic and Racial Studies* 30 (6), 1024–1054.

Wallace, C. (2005) Conversations around the literacy hour in a multilingual London primary school. *Language and Education* 19 (4), 322–338.

8 Becoming Biliterate Within the Crossroads of Home and School: Insights Gained From Taking Multiple Theoretical Stances

Bobbie Kabuto

Introduction

When my daughter Emma was six years old, I was invited to teach a graduate class about the Japanese writing system. Emma joined me and as soon as we went into the classroom she immediately went to the board to write in Japanese. Slightly taken aback by Emma's use of English and Japanese, a student in the class came up to me afterwards and asked, 'How did she learn to do that?' Before I could begin to provide an answer, Emma jumped in and said, 'Because I was born in Japan'.

How *do* young children become bilingual and biliterate individuals? I puzzled over this question for many years. From the time I was teaching second grade in a Japanese international school in Tokyo, I wondered how the children in my class and within the school could speak, read and write in not just two but sometimes three or more languages. With the birth of Emma in August 1998, I took a renewed interest in bilingualism and, as she began to pick up pens, pencils and crayons, her early biliteracy.

Researching Emma's paths into learning how to read and write in English and Japanese prompted me to go beyond the dominant cognitive and structural linguistic perspectives, particularly in the field of second language acquisition (SLA), and to acknowledge that singular theoretical frameworks provided incomplete pictures of the complexity of how children become biliterate within the home, school and community, particularly when there are ideological tensions among language use within and across those domains. Becoming biliterate is more than learning the forms and functions of two or more written languages; it means becoming someone in a world defined by conventional constraints related to the social, cultural and linguistic domains that languages embody. At the heart of the tension between what I was observing and documenting was acknowledging that language learning is more than the gradual accumulation and conversion of one form into another. How and what Emma learned when she learned to read and write in multiple languages could not be separated from the social, cultural, historical and political factors within which language was embedded.

In this chapter I take sociocultural, linguistic, semiotic and anthropological perspectives to discuss the complexity of becoming biliterate at the crossroads of home and school. I argue that interdisciplinary approaches to learning in multilingual literacies can create complementary frameworks that provide insights into how the local micro-aspects of written language are intricately intertwined with larger ideologies, sociocultural identities and spaces involving people, places, practices and things.

Learning involves tensions – not only in language forms, but also in who we think we are and who we want to become. To discuss these issues, I present a case study of my daughter, Emma, learning to become biliterate in the home and what occurred when learning in home and school collided. Elsewhere, I provide extensive discussions on Emma's learning to read and write in Japanese and English (Kabuto, 2008, 2010). For the purposes of this chapter, I spotlight Emma's bilingual writing practices. Across three sections I describe selected material, gathered from Emma's multilingual literacy practices, and interpret it by drawing on the explanatory theoretical perspectives of language and text, identity and language ideologies. I begin by presenting the case study and ethnographic methodology.

Becoming Biliterate – A Case Study

Emma was born in Tokyo, Japan, where we lived until she was two years, five months old. We then moved to a suburban, diverse community on the north shore of Long Island, New York. At the time of our move, the total population of our town was 15,215: 75.1% were white, 12.3% were African-American, 3.6% were Asian and 12.5% were Hispanic or Latino[1] (according to US census figures for 2006).

Emma attended the local preschool and a Japanese Saturday school from the age of three years. The decision to have her attend both schooling programmes was based on our wish to support her bilingualism and biliteracy. We knew that moving to New York would cause a switch in her language use to become English dominant, and our fear of her loss of ability to speak Japanese, in particular to be able to communicate with her Japanese grandparents, led her father, Jay, and I to search out resources to support our family's bilingual identity. After Emma finished preschool at five years old, she moved into the local public school. At the same time, she continued with Japanese school until she was nine years old.

The Japanese school was housed in the local middle school and attracted *chyuzain* families, or families who live abroad for work purposes. In a phenomenon similar to transnationalism, these families were sent to the USA by Japanese companies, which supported their work overseas for a period of five to seven years. Given the desire to closely follow the curriculum in schools in Japan, the Japanese government donated textbooks to Emma's Japanese school and children were taught in mathematics, Japanese social studies and Japanese language arts (*Kokugo*). Because of the pressure to keep up with a Japanese curriculum, Emma began to have a difficult time with the curricular demands of Japanese school, and as a result Jay and I decided to allow her to exit Japanese school at the end of third grade.

Data Collection

Data were collected when Emma was between the ages of three and seven. The sources used for this ethnographic study provided both qualitative and quantitative data. The qualitative data consisted of observational field notes and reflexive notes and the quantitative data included descriptive statistics on Emma's self-produced signs and on school documents from the public school only.

Qualitative data: Field notes and reflexive notes

Observational data of the social context for Emma's biliteracy learning were recorded in field notes. Daily field notes recorded a variety of literacy practices in which Emma participated in the home and community. In addition to observational notes, reflexive notes documented the ways in which my role as 'mother' and as 'researcher' informed this study (see Kabuto, 2008, for a discussion of parent research).

Reflexive notes, which documented my role by making it transparent in the research, also provided me with a venue for addressing ethical issues within the research. Using reflexivity to address ethical issues meant acknowledging Emma's voiced opinions about how I conducted the research. My positioning Emma as a 'co-researcher', as Christensen and Prout (2002) advocate, encouraged her to have a say in how and what I collected during the study. For instance, if Emma did not want me to audio-tape, I took notes. Other times, when Emma did not want me to keep the original writing artefact, I asked if I could photocopy it. My goal was to be respectful of Emma's private spaces but to maintain rigour and consistency in my data collection.

Quantitative data: Self-produced writing and drawing artefacts

A total of 372 Emma's artefacts were collected in the home between the ages three and seven (see Table 8.1). Between the ages of three and four, Emma's signs consisted of English (56.7%) and images (41.0%). A small

Table 8.1 Distribution of Emma's collected writing and drawing between three and seven years of age

Languages	Age (years; months)			
	3;0 – 3;11	4;0 – 4;11	5;0 – 5;11	6;0 – 6;11
English	56.7%	36.6%	58.7%	75.3%
Japanese	0	24.4%	31.7%	3.2%
English and Japanese	0.7%	3.7%	4.8%	0
Image-only	41.0%	35.4%	4.8%	21.5%
Language-like	0.7%	0	0	12.9%
Total number of artefacts	134	82	63	93

number of the artefacts were considered language-like (0.7%), as they were markings like wavy lines or letter-like symbols that demonstrated Emma's movement into conventional written language. By the time that Emma was between the ages of four and five, written Japanese began to appear regularly as a script choice in her writings. During this time, while drawings were a major meaning carrier, her incorporation of English decreased from the previous year. At five years old (during kindergarten), English and Japanese as script choices increased as images decreased, suggesting Emma's movement away from drawings to written language. However, between the ages of six and seven, Emma entered first grade, and there was a dramatic increase in her use of English and decrease in her use of Japanese. Only 3.2% of her artefacts during this time included written Japanese.

However from five to seven years of age, a shift in the content of Emma's writings and drawings occurred. Between the ages of five and six, 58.7% of Emma's artefacts were about herself and her family, while between six and seven years of age (first grade) there was another decrease in this content, to 37.8%. At the same time, between the ages of six and seven years, artefacts that represented school-based reading and writing practices emerged and represented 45.2% of the artefacts collected within that year. Emma wrote lists of short vowels or created a series of mathematical addition and/or subtraction sentences. This shift in content in Emma's writing and drawing in the home corresponded with an increase in the amount of school work that she completed and is illustrative the data collected from school documents.

School documents

School documents, collected only from the public school, consisted of report cards, homework and schoolwork that were sent home. These types of documents were distributed in a communication folder that came home at the end of each week. In kindergarten and first grade, parents received report cards in the autumn and spring. The report cards were composed of checklists, and teachers provided additional narrative comments about the individual subject areas. Documentation from parent–teacher conferences was added to this category.

Collecting the types and content of work done at school and sent home at the end of the week did not document the complete body of work that Emma did in school. It, however, captured a picture of what type of school work is communicated to parents. While Emma was in kindergarten, I collected 84 pieces of schoolwork, which formed two categories: commercially produced work and self-produced work (see Table 8.2). Work placed into the commercially produced category consisted of worksheets or workbook pages which focused on handwriting, letter formation, books, writing words and writing sentences. Within these subcategories, the largest percentage of work sent home was handwriting practice from a handwriting book. This subcategory was closely followed by worksheets that focused on letter and number formation. The smallest percentage of work consisted of writing words, followed by sentences.

Interestingly, the subcategories were sent home in a hierarchical fashion. The largest subcategories, handwriting and letter formation, were sent home first, that is, at the beginning of the school year, while the smallest subcategories, writing words and sentences, were sent home towards the end of the school year.

The second category comprised artefacts that Emma produced herself. The only type of work sent home within this category was journals for free writing (11.9%). Emma had a journal for each month of the school year and the teacher required the students to write in it once or twice a week. I received all of the journals together at the end of the school year.

During the first grade, the total number of pieces of schoolwork sent home drastically increased, to 562, of which 93.2% were commercially produced materials and 6.8% were self-created. Out of the 93.2%, 53.2% addressed English language arts and 40% were related to mathematics. Table 8.2 shows the breakdown of categories with corresponding percentages of work sent home within English language arts. The largest subcategory here was workbook pages that integrated writing and word matching. These workbook pages had one part in which the student had to write sentences using given words and another part in which students had to match words with pictures or definitions. The other percentages were spread across the other subcategories: filling in the blank (8.9%), following directions (3.6%), theme-related reading and writing (6.4%), reading comprehension (5.9%) and writing the alphabet (1.8%).

Again in the first grade, self-produced writing came in at only 6.8%, a much smaller percentage than the commercially produced writing materials. Unlike kindergarten, Emma's self-produced writing addressed only weekly spelling words or writing sentences. As part of the spelling curriculum, Emma was asked to use spelling words in sentences or to copy spelling words.

Table 8.2 Distribution of Emma's collected artefacts in kindergarten and first grade

Content	Commercial		Self-produced		Totals
	No. of artefacts	%	No. of artefacts	%	
Kindergarten					
Handwriting practice	29	34.5%	0	0%	
Writing numbers	3	3.6%	0	0%	
Writing the alphabet	18	21.4%	0	0%	
Books or journals	7	8.3%	10	11.9%	
Writing words	10	11.9%	0	0%	
Writing sentences	7	8.3%	0	0%	
Total	74		10		84
Total percentages*		88.1%		11.9%	100%
First grade					
Math worksheets	225	40.0%	0	0%	
English language arts	299	53.2%	38	6.8%	
Totals	524		38		562
Percentages		93.2%		6.8%	100%
Further breakdown of the English language arts work					
Fill in blanks	50	8.9%	0	0%	
Writing and matching words	151	26.9%	0	0%	
Worksheets that address following directions	20	3.6%	0	0%	
Sheets that addressed the classroom science or social studies theme	35	6.2%	0	0%	
Reading comprehension	33	5.9%	0	0%	
Writing alphabet letters	10	1.8%	0	0%	
Self-writing such as journals or sentences with spelling words	0	0%	38	6.8%	
Total artefacts from English language arts work	299		38		337
Total percentages* from English language arts work		53.2%		6.8%	60%

*Percentages may be approximate due to rounding up.

The narratives that arose through the juxtaposition of qualitative and quantitative data raised interesting and complex questions. I found myself asking questions such as: What purposes did writing in two languages and in multiple scripts serve for Emma? Why were there shifts in how she used written language in the home and school, and in how she viewed herself as a bilingual and biliterate child? What happened when Emma's bilingual and biliterate world met the monolingual institutional practices of school? In reading across the literature in the areas of semiotics, sociocultural theory, sociolinguistics and anthropology, I discovered that the data could not be pigeonholed into one framework rather than another, as each contributed to the data and findings.

Taking Multiple Theoretical Stances

The study began to form around three major connecting themes: language and text; socially constructed identities; and language ideologies. Around these three themes, four perspectives fed into the theoretical and the conceptual frameworks of the study.

Language and text

Language and text have social roots and are semiotic in nature. Taking a sociocultural perspective to language and learning, researchers following a Vygotskian perspective assert the sociocultural situatedness of learning; more specifically, learning is rooted in everyday social and cultural experiences (Gutierrez & Rogoff, 2003; Lave, 1988; Lave & Wenger, 1991; Moll, 1992). Within this perspective, human action is mediated by tools and signs such as spoken and written languages.

From a Vygotskian perspective, written language can serve as a cultural tool system that is 'oriented outward, toward the transformation of the physical and social reality' (Blanck in Vygotsky, 1986: 45), what Vygotsky describes as a 'technical tool'. As a technical tool, written language can serve an interpersonal function, developing social relationships and cultural worlds, which give meaning not only to written language, but also to the social roles that Emma participated in as she used written language (Wertsch, 1991). This is an idea to which I will return in my discussion of identity.

On the other hand, written language is a sign system, or what Vygotsky compared to a 'psychological tool', which can be used to transform individual learning through semiotic mediation. Vygotsky's major argument is that semiotic mediation has social origins. Vygotsky, however, did little to elaborate on the idea of semiotic mediation and what it would look like with written language.

Kress (1997) took a particular interest how children's literacy development can be understood through semiotic mediation, within the field of social semiotics. Kress's work emphasises that children create meaning through a range of media as they employ modes or an organised means of representation. According to semiotic perspectives, communication and the construction of meaning are always multimodal. While this may be the case, researchers contend that certain modes are privileged over others, particularly in schools. Kress suggests that children move from the multimodal world of learning in the home and community to the linear organisation of reading and writing in schools. The 'stuff' that children use to create meaning within their transactions with their social environments no longer counts in schools.

While Kress drew a linkage between the 'stuff' and the materials that children have available in their environment, bilingual children in particular may draw from other available resources, such as writing scripts. The work of Kenner and Kress (2003) and Kabuto (2010) illustrate how early biliterate children view scripts as modes.

Between the ages of three and six, Emma viewed both English and Japanese scripts as possibilities for communicating meaning. At three years old, her initial attempts at writing favoured English over Japanese. Also during this time, Emma used both English and Japanese scripts in her writing artefacts. As soon as she started writing, Emma did not necessarily see English and Japanese scripts as separate from one another. This characteristic continued through Emma's early years. Until the age of six, she would write in both systems. The ways in which Emma combined scripts, such as Japanese Hiragana with the English Roman alphabet, in her writing was the result her understanding of how scripts held communicational capacities that connected to the social worlds in which she participated and the people in those worlds (Kabuto, 2010). This position is very different from ones that view script-switching as a lack of knowledge in one language resulting in the language user supplementing it with another language. On the contrary, Emma's selection of scripts was the result of motivated action and reaction to the people and places around her.

Scripts allowed her to create a social and cultural reality and actively transform the social spaces in which she participated. For example, Emma at the age of five years and months created a birthday card for her friend Erika from Japanese school. Erika's birthday party was on Valentine's Day, prompting Emma to write 'Happy Valentine's Day' (with my assistance on spelling) on the front of the card. Emma then wrote 'From Emma [to] Erika' in Hiragana. Noting that Emma could have written 'Happy Valentine's Day' in Japanese – it is celebrated in Japan and in her Japanese school – I asked Emma why she wrote in Japanese and English. She replied that she needed to write Happy Valentine's Day in English because she 'lives in America' and the greeting in Japanese because Erika is Japanese. Through the employment of Japanese- and English-based scripts, Emma created a bilingual and biliterate world and could engage in that world in an authentic manner through her relationships with other people.

The multimodal nature of Emma's early writing did not lie just in written language systems, but also in her consistent use of other modes, such as images. Between the ages of three and five, Emma mostly drew pictures or wrote about herself and her family. The literature on early writing indicates that it evolves out of children's fundamental desire to understand their sense of self, or who they are in relation to other people (Baghban, 2007). Cards, poems, landscapes and portraits were among the many artefacts that Emma created during this time. In addition, as people entered Emma's life (such as with the birth of her brother Rick), they became the object or audience of her writings and drawings.

At the same time, the quantitative data highlight interesting shifts in the percentages and content of Emma's writing at home and at school. Considering Emma's home and school artefacts together suggests that the more Emma participated in school, the more her writing began to shift in the home to look like her school writing. She used less written Japanese in the home and more English. Table 8.1 shows that between the ages of three and six, Emma's uses of Japanese increased each year, but then dramatically decreased between the ages of six and seven (31.7% to 3.2%), when she went from kindergarten to first grade. Between the ages of four and seven there was a consistent increase in her use of English, and by the time she was seven 75.3% of her writing in the home used only English.

Over the four years of this study, Emma's uses of written language within her textual artefacts changed as she entered into different types of social domains, in particular the movement from preschool to kindergarten to first grade. Scripts as semiotic and technical tools are oriented outwards, towards social contexts that give meaning to those scripts and the person creating them. In essence, by engaging in writing, Emma was actively creating an identity through her self-in-action, and by actively employing scripts she could work through the multiple ideological stances and meaning potentials that scripts hold in understanding and engaging in the social domains in which she participated (Holland et al., 1998; Rowsell & Pahl, 2007).

Identities

Language and text are also sites for identity work. Mikhail Bakhtin (1981) is one of the fundamental theorists who argue that language and text are dialogic, meaning that there are always at least two voices: the voice of the speaker and the voice of the persons being addressed. The interaction between these voices assists in the development of identity as we align with the responses of others in our environment, either directly or by presupposing their voices. Bakhtin suggested that texts are spaces where one attempts to orchestrate the multiple voices, leading to his concept of 'self-authoring'.

Language and texts are also connected to social and cultural domains and structures. Therefore the scripts become part of what Gee (1996) describes as a 'toolkit' from which bilingual children select to align themselves or to challenge the social domains within which the text is embedded. In other words, bilingual children have the potential to select written languages from their toolkit in the process of self-authoring as they actively engage in writing. The work in anthropology on semiotics advances our understanding of how the situated selection of scripts is indexical of social identity. Of particular interest is work deriving from the writings of Charles Sanders Peirce on semiotics.

Peirce's semiotic model (Buchler, 1955) emphasises that a sign is developed from a triadic relationship composed of: a sign, an object and an interpretant. A sign within this triadic relationship is defined as something that stands for its object and is itself composed of three modes: an icon, an index and a symbol. Peirce proposed that the essence of written language represents a symbolic mode because symbolic modes are governed by social conventions. While this may be the case, research in linguistics and linguistic anthropology suggests that written language can also move between iconic and indexical modes. The classic example provided by researchers involves a proper name, and Emma's own understanding of her name illustrates how she could use it to position herself and construct identities within home and school.

Emma's name is both an Anglophone and a Japanese name. Because Jay and I were cognizant of how personal names create cultural identities, we decided to give Emma a name that would 'sound' both English and Japanese and could be represented in both orthographies. Table 8.3 shows Emma's name written in each script related to English and Japanese, and it also represents Emma's name in its symbolic mode, which is defined as the mode composed of conventional, rule-governed characteristics. In other words, 'Emma' written in the Roman alphabet has rule-governed characters, as does 'Emma' written in the Japanese Hiragana script. 'Emma' written in the Roman alphabet, however, in its indexical mode may point to a different meaning than 'Emma' written in Japanese Hiragana, or even in Chinese Kanji. In its indexical mode, a name in a particular script may point to, or index, other social meanings or structures, particularly because without the interaction of the social there cannot be meaning; it is the social structure that frames how meanings are understood, interpreted and/or negotiated. In essence, language is indexical of social and cultural identities and, as

Table 8.3 Emma's name in Japanese and English scripts

English, Roman	Japanese, Hiragana	Japanese, Katakana	Japanese, Roman	Japanese, Kanji
Emma	えま	エマ	Ema	絵馬

such, Emma's name became a critical way for her to position herself both in school and at home.

During her kindergarten year, Emma wrote her name in both English and Hiragana on 35% of her school artefacts. One night, when I observed Emma writing her name in English and Japanese on a phonics homework sheet, I questioned her actions. She replied, 'I am the only one who knows Japanese, so no one will know what I am writing but me'. One of many other similar comments, Emma's reflection of her actions suggests her understanding of how name writing both includes and excludes oneself from participatory spaces. Within any written or spoken text there are sediments of identity, and in this example the phonics worksheet, with juxtaposition of Emma's name in both English and Japanese with the phonics content, there are sediments of her identity that assist in recreating the purpose of the worksheet for Emma (Rowsell & Pahl, 2007).

Of additional interest to this study were the ways in which bilingual writing embodies cultural tools and symbols and are mediational in situated, socially constructed 'selves' and identities over time. In particular, 'selves' are socially constructed through the medium of language and text (Fairclough, 1995, 2001; Ivanic, 1988). Thus, language and text are seen foremost as cultural tool systems that have the possibility to transform one's self-in-practice and to mediate the social environment. Both have social semiotic roots and are bound with meaning (Halliday, 1993).

In the home, Emma's belief was that the use of two written languages allowed her to identify with her Japanese- and/or English-speaking friends and family. Similarly, she may have written in Japanese to identify with Japanese childhood practices, and in English for American ones. Weighing the available writing possibilities that were accessible to her, Emma selected those that would best address the person to whom she was writing within the larger societal context (Kabuto, 2010). In this way, Emma acknowledged that writing in two languages held the potential to maintain social relationships.

Emma's kindergarten and first-grade years saw a shift in her bilingual-script writing. In the home, as mentioned above, none of her self-produced artefacts included two languages, and only 3.2% included Japanese. The number of school artefacts drastically increased from 84 pieces in kindergarten to 562 in the first grade. In addition, Emma's desire to write her name in Japanese and English on her first-grade work ceased, as none of her papers sent home had her name written in both languages. Noticing this change, I asked Emma (then aged six years and two months) why she no longer wrote her name in Japanese in school. 'I don't want to. This is America. You speak English in America. Everyone speaks English in America', Emma replied. I replied that she speaks Japanese in Japanese school. Emma quickly responded, 'Japanese school is in New York and New York is in America'. Emma's father entered into the conversation to remind her that we use both languages in our home. 'Our home is in New York and New York is American. I want to speak English', Emma reiterated. Her comments indicated tensions in her beliefs about language use. While she did not completely abandon her use of Japanese – she was still attending Japanese school and was a member of a family who used both languages regularly inside and outside the home – her actions suggest that she was not completely complacent in accepting beliefs about how and when one should act with and through language. Emma's actions through writing and talking illustrate how she actively engaged in debates within her developing identities and how her identities were associated with larger belief systems, in particular language ideologies.

Language ideologies

Sociolinguistics and linguistic anthropology have created a bridge between micro-sociolinguistics, the study of language at the discourse level, and macro-sociolinguistics, the ways in which languages index multiple role relationships and are used as a social mechanism for the negotiation and creation of social roles and networks (Auer, 1999; Li Wei, 2000). In particular, language use is described as verbal action in the realms of identity and power relationships (Auer, 1999). Research on bilingualism and biliteracy has highlighted the relationships between language learning and social and cultural processes (e.g. Hornberger, 2000; Perez, 2004). Among these social processes, the critical examination of language ideologies, or unexamined beliefs of language use, has been a fruitful of enquiry (Woolard, 1998; Woolard & Schieffelin, 1994). Researchers have studied how language ideologies mediate language choice among children in bilingual classrooms (Martinez-Roldan & Malave, 2004; Volk & Angelova, 2007) and homes (Martinez-Roldan & Malave, 2004).

Researchers have argued that language ideologies are 'mediating discourses between social groups and the ways they use language' (Volk & Angelova, 2007: 179). For instance, the movement toward English-only learning in schools in the USA contends that the only acceptable way to educate linguistically diverse children is through the medium of English (Auerbach, 1993). Consequently, with this approach, the use of English and that of languages other than English come into conflict.

Beliefs about language are tied to what Gee (1996) refers to as primary and secondary Discourse (with a capital 'D') communities. For children, the home is a primary Discourse community because it is where children are socialised into 'initial taken-for-granted understandings of who we are and who people "like us" are' (Gee, 1996: 137). Children like Emma, who are raised in linguistically diverse homes, recognise the importance of their native languages in connecting themselves with family and community, and this recognition is the result of children being active members in homes and communities around literacy. They interact with multiple written languages in the home and may participate in different book-reading events, with storybooks, activity books or religious texts in different languages (Gregory *et al.*, 2004; Kabuto, 2010).

At the same time, young bilingual children go to school and learn the dominant language of the community. For instance, Gregory (1996) studied children's interactions with religious texts such as the Koran in London and found that children not only develop an awareness of the nature of written language but also acquire particular daily routines around texts. The social routines were just as important to reading but were not always recognised within schools. Consequently, such a child's primary Discourse becomes connected to valuing the ways in which multiple written languages can allow the child to be an engaged member of his or her home and community.

Yet as linguistically diverse children venture out of the home, their language beliefs come into contact with other secondary Discourse communities, such as educational institutions. In the process of language contact, different ideologies compete because they are closely linked to power. The goal of ideological contestation is to sustain particular power relationships and, more specifically, to maintain unequal power relationships (Fairclough, 2001; Tollefson, 1991). There is also a power contained *within* language ideologies to shift young children's choices about how and when to use multiple written languages, which leads researchers to argue that ideologies are 'power-linked discourses' (Woolard, 1998: 7).

Writing can be liberating, meaning that individuals use writing to create a voice to express ideas that are meaningful to themselves (Giroux, 1983). This liberation is connected to human agency (Holland *et al.*, 1998). Writing allows individuals to express their opinions and viewpoints in their own voices; it has the capability to challenge unexamined beliefs about society and language. Young biliterate children can convey their thoughts and impressions of the world through multiple written languages and at the same time challenge English as the privileged medium of written communication in certain social contexts.

For instance, three months into kindergarten, Emma (aged five years and three months) asked her father to play sumo wrestling, her favourite game at the time. Each took opposing stances and placed one fist on the ground to charge after the cue *take no okota* was given. Listening from the next room, I heard Emma begging to play the game one more time: 'Please, daddy. One time.' Then Emma said, 'Daddy, I don't want to be Japanese anymore'. Jay replied, 'Soo. [Really.] Zyaa, sumo shiyo. [Okay. Let's play sumo wrestling.]' Not responding directly to Emma's comment about her not wanting 'to be Japanese anymore', Jay decided to give into Emma's request to play sumo wrestling. When I later asked Jay about Emma's comment and how he felt about it, he shrugged it off, feeling that it was a passing feeling for her. Interestingly, it was. Three months later, in January, Emma started writing her name in Japanese and English on her school work, in part as a presentation of herself as a biliterate child. Furthermore, in kindergarten I collected the largest percentage of Japanese writing artefacts (31.7%) among the four years of the collection process.

While there were times when Emma challenged her bilingual and biliterate behaviours, her writing behaviours in the home and at school contradicted this comment in kindergarten. By writing in two languages, Emma seemed to acknowledge that language provided her with power within the social structures within which her writing was embedded. In the home, the integration of English and Japanese was a way of writing relationships with other people and connecting to different types of social practices, such as celebrating Valentine's Day or birthdays. In school, Emma viewed the use of multiple scripts, in some way, as challenging the mono-lingual practices of school.

Emma's teachers' responses or lack of responses to her biliterate behaviours also began to shape her beliefs about language use. At parent–teacher conferences, I discovered that Emma's teacher was aware of her actions and described her behaviour as 'refreshing'. Her teacher appeared to enjoy watching Emma writing in multiple scripts, although she did not fully encourage it in the classroom. The teacher did not acknowledge Emma's biliterate behaviours on report cards or in other types of formal documents. The teacher's main comment on her report card related to Emma's successful adjustment to kindergarten, which was partly related to her ability to use English in a manner appropriate for a child at the same the age and grade. Emma's teacher's description of her biliterate behaviours as 'refreshing' may have encouraged Emma to demonstrate them more in school. At the same time, the teacher did not mind because her biliterate behaviours did not interfere with the use of English as the dominant language practice in school.

Unlike Emma's kindergarten teacher, her first-grade teacher was not aware of her biliterate behaviours. During the end-of-the-year conference, when we were given a written report, the teacher said that she did not write or speak in Japanese. Because Emma did not exhibit biliterate behaviours in the classroom, her teacher did not know the extent of her Japanese abilities. In the teacher's written report, in which she noted that Emma was a confident writer who used sight vocabulary and phonetic spellings and who wrote with central ideas, Emma was commended for her increasing English writing proficiency. Emma's teacher felt that she was an asset to the class and a hard worker. Emma's teacher applauded her as an English-dominant speaker, reader and writer. Sensing her teacher's appreciation of her English ability, Emma began to shift her beliefs of herself as a bilingual child to a monolingual child. Incidentally, in her first-grade year, Emma produced the least number of Japanese artefacts, began supporting the belief that English should be the dominant language inside and outside the home, and created artefacts that mirrored school-based writing practices.

During the first five years of her life, Emma learned and appreciated how the ability to write in two languages provided her with access to a variety of social groups as they created and maintained social relationships with others. Yet these beliefs and her consequent behaviours came to a sudden stop in first grade. In addition to shifts in her written language choices, there were also changes in the content of the writing artefacts that she produced in the home.

Emma voraciously created artefacts such as school-like worksheets in the home. She graded self-created worksheets with an A+ or an F. She also developed worksheets for imaginary people, such as Cinderella. The content of these writing pieces was consistent with the types of work brought home from school. Out of the 562 pieces of work that were sent home in first grade, 40% of the worksheets were mathematics sheets. The second largest category were worksheets that addressed individual words (26.9%) through activities such as writing rhyming words or circling the words with the same vowel sound.

While first grade saw a substantial decrease in Emma's writing in Japanese, it was also a time when school-based reading and writing practices entered into Emma's writing in the home. Emma appeared to develop strong school-based connections to English and to being a first-grade student 'in America', as she put it. Within this process, Emma reproduced particular language ideologies that contradicted what it means to be bilingual and biliterate.

When Emma brought multiple ideological stances related to language in school, ideologies began to compete. Through the medium of writing, she evaluated them and placed social values on ideologies associated with home and with school. In essence, I argue that the evaluation occurred through Emma's motivated actions. Writing in different languages across a variety of social contexts, she evaluated other people's reactions, or lack thereof, to her bilingual writing. The evaluation process was an active one that involved assigning symbolic values not just to language. But it also required Emma to understand how languages are connected to social identities and power (Bourdieu, 1991; Kress & Hodge, 1979).

The movement from a bilingual home to a monolingual school came at a time when Emma reinvented herself. By reinventing herself through writing, she allowed the monolingual ideology to begin to dominate, and it eventually dominated across home and school contexts. From Emma's shifting uses of language in her writing, we could conclude that by the time she entered the first grade, she placed more social value on English, which affected the micro-level of discourse forms and function. At the same time, she built the substance of her writing by acting like a 'student' in her use of English and emulating the types of work that she was assigned and completed in school.

Shifts to English and representing school-based literacy practices were windows into how she attributed access to academic social structures and identities to the ability to speak and write in English. However, it counter-acted the process of learning to become bilingual and biliterate. Holland *et al.* write, 'Humans' capacity for self-objectification – and, through ob-jectification, for self-direction – plays into both their domination by social relations of power and their possibilities for (partial) liberation from these forces' (Holland *et al.*, 1998: 5). Emma's attempts at self-objectification surfaced through the medium of her bilingual writing, which allowed her to represent who she is or her multiple identities related to language. From kindergarten onwards, she quickly recognised that English was the language of power; it was a way of getting things done in school. Subsequently, the appearance of Emma's bilingual writing at school during this time also constituted an act of liberation from those hidden power structures related to language. She could challenge monolingual ideologies related to language and schooling. This means that Emma exercised more agency in voicing her language-related identities when she allowed herself to write in multiple languages. In other words, writing in English and Japanese served multiple roles for Emma. It was an act of agency and an act of social and linguistic reproduction within the first two years of schooling.

Combining People, Places, Practices and Things Across Disciplines

Emma constructed herself by learning to be a participating member in literacy events and their associated literacy practices within social worlds. Becoming biliterate involves developing relationships with other people through written language. It also involves writing within a variety of social contexts and structures, and sometimes those structures may have competing values on written language forms. Becoming biliterate also involves 'the things' or tools that are within one's toolkit. 'The things' in Emma's toolkit consisted of access to multiple scripts in two writing systems. These represented collective tools rather than separate tools. This concept of collective tools also metaphorically refers to patterns of choices available to Emma. It is important to note that not everyone has the same access to the same tools and no one person will have the same toolkit as the next. Furthermore, certain tools may have a higher status than others. The contestation of tools within toolkits can provide insights into how Emma employed the tools she had available to her and how they positioned her within social activities.

Controlling the interrelationships of the people, places and things is what becoming biliterate entails. And the addition of each theoretical perspective within the study of language, text, identity and ideology in learning to become biliterate began to close the gap by starting with the social activity (and cultural tools) and tracing its development back to the particulars of language and text within the home and school.

The combination of theoretical perspectives informed by each discipline presented in this chapter suggests the ways in which learning to read and write in two languages intersects with identity and language ideologies. The overarching framework centred writing as sociocultural, semiotic tools with which Emma created possibilities for self-hood, to challenge and reproduce language ideologies in a variety of practices at home and at school. To do so, learning to write in two languages involved the examination of writing as semiotic and social processes to understand how dominant ideologies constrained Emma's sense of self and, at the same time, challenged and liberated Emma's sense of self through tensions between 'self' and 'other', to redefine alternative selves. Consequently, language and text can be viewed as shaping and being shaped by identities and language ideologies situated in social, cultural and political contexts within which Emma was learning to read and write in English and Japanese, at the crossroads of home and school.

Conclusion

At the beginning of this chapter, I proposed that the movement across diverse fields of enquiry can create complementary frameworks that result in paradigm shifts, shifts that allow researchers and scholars to see data in new and productive ways. By describing how bilingualism has been traditionally studied as an example of how what we see is always framed by particular paradigms, I argued that the interpretations of data and findings are reflective of meta-theories underlying fields of study. My justification for shifting paradigms is that a singular field of study is insufficient to provide comprehensive explanations of the complexity of language, text, individual and social activity. Naturally, accounting for everything is an enormous task, but the more researchers and scholars begin to expand their analytical perspectives, the more they enrich theory through the incorporation of different types of knowledge related to other fields.

By applying this argument to a study of early biliteracy, we can see how a young bilingual and biliterate child engaged in the inherent complexity of learning to write is a social life bound by meaning. By juxtaposing frameworks, themes emerged across disciplines that, when combined, generated linkages. These linkages, then, formed complementary perspectives that held the possibility of filling in what was lacking in another theory. In turn, the complementary theoretical frameworks allowed for comprehensive understandings that tied the local written language production to larger sociocultural processes in becoming biliterate at the crossroads of home and school. Learning to become biliterate necessitates learning the writing forms that correspond to spoken languages, and yet these forms cannot be isolated from the context of social life. Bilingual writing is also indexical of social and cultural identities and power relationships.

Movements in education to standardise what we know and how we express what we know should compel educators to become interdisciplinary researchers. It seems that the more we know about the uncontrollable nature of language and literacy, the more policy-makers want to control it. Eliminating languages other than English in schools in the USA are ideological movements imbued with power and status. The tools that we use to teach in schools should not be separated from their theoretical underpinnings of learning, whose conceptual understandings are informed by a variety of disciplines. The challenges facing educators today are not necessarily how to teach language and literacy in schools, it is how to free ourselves from the ideological constraints that control how and what we teach in schools.

Note

1   Percentages equal 108.5% due to the US census data collected in categories described as 'White persons' rather than 'White, Not Hispanic persons'.

References

Auer, P. (1999) Introduction: Bilingual conversation revisited. In P. Auer (ed.) *Code-Switching in Conversation* (pp. 1–25). Florence, KY: Routledge.

Auerbach, E.R. (1993) Reexamining English only in ESL classrooms. *TESOL Quarterly* 27 (1), 9–32.

Baghban, M. (2007) Scribbles, labels, and stories: The role of drawing in the development of writing. *Young Children* 60 (1), 20–26.

Bakhtin, M.M. (1981) *The Dialogic Imagination: Four Essays by M.M. Bakhtin*.Austin, TX: University of Texas Press.

Bourdieu, P. (1991) *Language and Symbolic Power*. Cambridge, MA: Harvard University Press.

Buchler, J. (ed.) (1955) *Philosophical Writings of Peirce*. New York: Dover Publications.

Christensen, P. and Prout, A. (2002) Working with ethnical symmetry in social research with children. *Childhood* 9 (4), 477–497.

Fairclough, N. (1995) *Critical Discourse Analysis: The Critical Study of Language*. New York: Longman.

Fairclough, N. (2001) *Language and Power* (2nd edn). New York: Pearson.

Gee, J.P. (1996) *Social Linguistics and Literacies: Ideology and Discourse* (2nd edn). Philadelphia, PA: Routledge-Falmer.

Giroux, H. (1983) Ideology and agency in the process of schooling. *Journal of Education* 165 (1), 12–34.

Gregory, E. (1996) *Making Sense of a New World: Learning to Read in a Second Language*. London: Paul Chapman Publishing.

Gregory, E., Long, S. and Volk, D. (2004) A sociocultural approach to learning. In E. Gregory, S. Long and D. Volk (eds) *Many Pathways to Literacy: Young Children Learning With Siblings, Grandparents, Peers and Communities* (pp. 6–20). New York: Routledge-Falmer.

Gutierrez, K. and Rogoff, B. (2003) Cultural ways of learning: Individual traits of repertoires of practice. *Educational Researcher* 32 (5), 19–25.

Halliday, M.A.K. (1993) Towards a language-based theory of learning. *Linguistics and Education* 5, 93–116.

Holland, D., Lachicotte, W., Skinner, D. and Cain, C. (1998) *Identity and Agency in Cultural Worlds*. Cambridge, MA: Harvard University Press.

Hornberger, N. (2000) Multilingual literacies, literacy practices, and the continua of biliteracy. In M. Martin-Jones and K. Jones (eds) *Multilingual Literacies* (Vol. 10) (pp. 353–367). Amsterdam, PA: John Benjamins.

Ivanic, R. (1988) *Writing and Identity: The Discoursal Construction of Identity in Academic Writing*. Philadelphia, PA: John Benjamins.

Kabuto, B. (2008) Parent-research as a process of inquiry: An ethnographic perspective. *Ethnography and Education* 3 (2), 177–194.

Kabuto, B. (2010) Bilingual script writing as an act of identity. *Bilingual Research Journal* 33 (2), 130–149.

Kenner, C. and Kress, G. (2003) The multisemiotic resources of biliterate children. *Journal of Early Childhood Literacy* 3 (2), 179–202.

Kress, G. (1997) *Before Writing: Rethinking the Paths to Literacy*. New York: Routledge.

Kress, G. and Hodge, R. (1979) *Language as Ideology*. London: Routledge and Kegan Paul.

Lave, J. (1988) *Cognition in Practice*. New York: Cambridge University Press.

Lave, J. and Wenger, E. (1991) *Situated Learning: Legitimate Peripheral Participation*. New York: Cambridge University Press.

Martinez-Roldan, C. and Malave, G. (2004) Language ideologies mediating literacy and identity in bilingual context. *Journal of Early Childhood Literacy* 4 (2), 155–180.

Moll, L. (1992) Funds of knowledge for teaching: Using a qualitative approach to connect homes and classrooms. *Theory Into Practice* 31 (2), 132–141.

Perez, B. (2004) Language, literacy, and biliteracy. In B. Perez (ed.) *Sociocultural Contexts of Language and Literacy* (2nd edn) (pp. 25–56). Hillsdale, NJ: Erlbaum.

Rowsell, J. and Pahl, K. (2007) Sedimented identities in texts: Instances of practice. *Reading Research Quarterly* 42 (3), 388–404.

Tollefson, J. (1991) *Planning Language, Planning Inequality*. New York: Longman.

Volk, D. and Angelova, M. (2007) Language ideology and the mediation of language choice in peer interactions in a dual-language first grade. *Journal of Language, Identity, and Education* 6(3), 177–199.

Vygotsky, L. (1986) *Thought and Language*. Cambridge, MA: MIT Press.

Li Wei (2000) Dimensions of bilingualism. In L. Wei (ed.) *The Bilingualism Reader* (pp. 3–25). New York: Routledge.

Wertsch, J. (1991) *Voices of the Mind*. Hemel Hempstead: Harvester Wheatsheaf.

Woolard, K. (1998) Language ideology as a field of inquiry. In B. Schieffelin, K. Woolard and K. Paul (eds) *Language Ideologies: Practice and Theory* (pp. 3–47). New York: Oxford University Press.

Woolard, K. and Schieffelin, B. (1994) Language ideology. *Annual Review of Anthropology* 23, 55–82.

Index